MEN AND THEIR MOTIVES

Founded by C. K. Ogden

The International Library of Psychology

GENERAL PSYCHOLOGY
In 38 Volumes

MEN AND THEIR MOTIVES

Psycho-Analytical Studies

J C FLUGEL

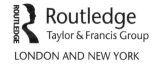

Routledge
Taylor & Francis Group

LONDON AND NEW YORK

First published in 1934 by
Routledge and Kegan Paul Ltd
2 Park Square, Milton Park, Abingdon, Oxfordshire OX14 4RN
711 Third Avenue, New York, NY 10017

First issued in paperback 2014

Routledge is an imprint of the Taylor and Francis Group, an informa business

British Library Cataloguing in Publication Data
A CIP catalogue record for this book
is available from the British Library

Men and their Motives
ISBN 978-0415-21016-4
General Psychology: 38 Volumes
ISBN 0415-21129-8
The International Library of Psychology: 204 Volumes
ISBN 0415-19132-7

ISBN 13: 978-1-138-88244-7 (pbk)
ISBN 13: 978-0-415-21016-4 (hbk)

CONTENTS

PREFACE

OF the eight essays which compose this book, six have been reprinted, with some additions and alterations, from the *British Journal of Medical Psychology*, the *International Journal of Psycho-analysis* and the *Psychoanalytic Quarterly*. We are greatly obliged to the editors of these periodicals for permission to include them in the present collection. Of the remaining two, one—that on " The Psychology of Birth Control "—is in part a modification of an article in the *British Journal of Medical Psychology* and is in part new, while the other—that on " Jealousy "—has not before been published.

Men and their Motives

THE PSYCHOLOGY OF BIRTH CONTROL

I. *The General Attitude to Birth Control and Neo-Malthusianism.*
II. *Some Unconscious Motives in the Opponents of Birth Control.*
III. *Some Unconscious Motives in the Supporters of Birth Control.*

I

THE GENERAL ATTITUDE TO BIRTH CONTROL AND NEO-MALTHUSIANISM

BIRTH control has had a curious and fluctuating history. The necessity for some control of population had often been recognized implicitly (and doubtless here and there explicitly) since the earliest times, especially among peoples whose geographical or political situation prevented the occupation of fresh territory as their numbers increased. Such control was partly exercised by the method of infanticide, though social customs limiting in one way or another the amount of sexual intercourse have always played some part. It may be that some methods of contraception were known to primitive peoples. All we are sure of, however, is that in the eighteenth century certain of the mechanical methods still in use were beginning to find favour at any rate among a few of the upper classes in Europe. On the theoretical side the greatest event was the publication of Malthus's *Essay on the Principles of Population* in 1798. Malthus herein stated the funda-

A 1

mental law that, as in the case of other animals, so too in man, the reproductive powers are greatly in excess of the actual possibilities of increase as determined by the amount of food available—a law that has ever since met with a most varied reception. Hailed by some as the most important proposition in sociology and economics, it has always encountered hedging or open opposition on the part of others; so much so that, even to-day, more than 130 years after its formulation, it cannot be said to be generally accepted, much less satisfactorily refuted. This ambiguous attitude is all the more remarkable in that both Darwin and Wallace were led to their ideas of evolution through their reading of Malthus, whose biological doctrine forms indeed one of the essential elements of Darwin's theory. Darwinism has—in its main outlines, if not in its detailed formulations—been accepted now for many years, but that part of the whole which constituted the first step in Darwin's own argument still receives a dubious welcome—a curious and illogical state of affairs which seems to indicate that there are perhaps some special psychological difficulties in the way of its acceptance.

We have said that Malthus's *Essay* was an event on the theoretical side, for of course Malthus never recommended birth control, which would have come under his category of 'vice.' For Malthus there was no alternative to the miseries of over-population but late marriage and the sexual abstinence that this implied. It was not till the second half of the nineteenth century that there arose the school of so-called neo-Malthusianism which was bold enough to propose a method of enjoying the pleasures of sex while escaping from the penalties of poverty. Although the Malthusian doctrine had in the meantime to some extent been incorporated into orthodox economics by a no less influential writer than J. S. Mill (not to speak of others), the neo-Malthusians remained for many years a relatively small body who gained few avowed adherents, and this in spite of the immense advertisement given to their cause by the prosecution of Bradlaugh and Mrs. Besant for the diffusion of a birth control pamphlet in 1877. Nevertheless, statistics indicate that the *practice* of birth control has made continual strides ever since that date,[1] for in the immediately following years the birth-rates of most civilized countries began to fall and have gone on falling to this day. The continued drop in human fertility, as indicated by these figures, represents perhaps one of the most remarkable changes in human life—and has indeed been regarded by some, with much show of reason, as a turning point in human history. Nevertheless, comparatively little notice was taken of the strange phenomenon. By the great majority it was vaguely deplored as a social evil, by the very few up-holders of neo-Malthusianism it was regarded as a hopeful sign of better times. Following the Great War, a changed attitude was manifested by the intellectuals, who began to come out definitely in favour of birth control, while one or two heroic workers—notably Marie Stopes in England and Margaret Sanger in America — set the fashion for open help and propaganda on the practical side. As a result of this work and discussion on the part of a relatively few influential people, the limitation of population by means of birth

---

[1] Marie Stopes in her *Contraception ; its Theory, History and Practice* (p. 306, 3rd ed.), suggests that in reality the fall in the birth-rate, due to the use of contraceptive measures, had begun before this, but is masked in the official figures by the fact that the registration of births only became compulsory (and therefore complete) at about the same time.

control (or contraception, as it should more properly be called) is no longer an almost completely neglected subject, as it was for many years before the war, but is one that has at least been heard of by the vast majority of civilized people. Birth control has in recent years become a subject which is recognized to have important social bearings.

But this increased attention to the existence and possibilities of birth control has brought comparatively little clarification of the reasons why it is desirable or undesirable. The intellectuals, who are mainly responsible for the greater publicity given to the subject, have tended to take the benefits of birth control for granted, without any very deep discussion of the reasons that may have led them to their advocacy of the practice. Even the writers on the economic and racial aspects of population have often contrived to write learned articles and volumes without very clearly or definitely committing themselves as to the truth or falsity of Malthus's law. Meanwhile, the leaders of reaction and the vast masses who vaguely follow them have tightened their attitude in face of the increasing power of their adversaries, but, apart from this, continue to use the same appeals and arguments that were in vogue at the beginning of the century and earlier. Few, if any, new objections seem to have been found; the undesirability or immorality of birth control is taken as more or less self-evident, though sterner measures have been resorted to for preventing the dissemination of birth control information, in the hope of discouraging its practice—notably in France, Italy and Ireland. These measures, however, have met with but indifferent success, and it is pretty clear that both in the three countries named and in many others there are great numbers of people who still practise birth control for private reasons but who have an uncomfortable feeling that they are committing an anti-social act in doing so.

Both among the supporters and among the opponents of birth control there would seem, therefore, to be some considerable degree of conflict—some real difficulty in facing, fairly and squarely, the question of the ultimate social value of birth control. With the exception of a few avowed neo-Malthusians, the supporters tend to shirk consideration of what—if true—must surely be its ultimate and most fundamental justification, *i.e.* Malthus's law, while its opponents take refuge in what are pretty clearly nothing but moral or political rationalizations (for the most part very emotionally coloured). Now, whether we look upon birth control as a striking cultural achievement or as a moral and political disaster, there is no one who denies that it is sociologically important. A psychological investigation of the motives that determine the public attitude to the subject can, therefore, scarcely fail to be of interest. The motives in question reveal themselves as in some respects unexpectedly complex—and even so our analysis can by no means be regarded as final or complete. We shall, moreover, confine ourselves to *motives* of the less logical and conscious sort, as distinct from *reasons* based on more or less objective evidence. It is not our business, therefore, to consider the law of Malthus, in its biological and economic bearings, as affording the ultimate justification of birth control, nor the merits and defects of sexual abstinence or sexual 'perversion' as possible alternatives. Nor shall we enter into such subsidiary but still highly important problems as those concerned with the connection between contraceptive methods and neurosis or other forms of disease, or with the eugenic bearings of birth control as it affects races, classes or individuals. We shall not even deal with the obvious fact of the immediate inconvenience and expense of most of the available methods of contraception. These are matters which can be dealt with on the basis of scientific evidence which falls outside the province of psychology. We are concerned here, rather, with the dimmer prejudices, feelings and convictions which make the impartial weighing of evidence upon these subjects a matter of difficulty and distaste.

Ideally, one who approaches such a task should himself have an open mind on the objective merits of the question in dispute. Unfortunately, such an ideal is itself difficult to realize. The psychologist who undertakes the examination of the attitude of others towards any social problem has usually (in the absence of any ulterior incentive) a keen belief in the importance of this problem. This implies almost inevitably that he has himself examined the objective aspects of the problem (though, of course, in the light of his own private prejudices), and has taken up some definite attitude with regard to it. In such a case it is perhaps best that he should confess this attitude frankly to begin with; not in order that he may feel himself absolved from the duty of trying to be unbiassed in his psychological investigation, but (as a friendly critic of the present writer once put it in relation to another matter) in order that the reader may make some correction for error. Now, in relation to this subject of birth control, I have to admit that I was convinced (on what I supposed to be objective grounds) of the fundamental truth of Malthus's law and of the desirability of contraception as a method of avoiding the evils to which it points, long before I attempted a psychological examination of the factors that determine people's attitude towards neo-Malthusianism. Indeed, this examination, when it was made, was to a large extent motivated by a desire to account for the fact that so many others had experienced difficulties in appreciating what seemed to me the extremely cogent evidence in favour of this doctrine. Not unnaturally, under these circumstances, the examination was primarily directed to the nature of the psychological factors that tend to cause a rejection of neo-Malthusianism on other than truly objective grounds.

My presupposition of the ultimate correctness of the neo-Malthusian view still to some extent colours the whole discussion,[1] but even (as I still cannot easily imagine) if this presupposition is unjustified, this does not mean that the psychological diagnosis of the opposition to birth control is necessarily in error. It must be admitted that (fortunately for humanity) it is possible to come to right decisions on false grounds; similarly, the grounds on which one refuses to give assent to a faulty proposition may themselves be false—and this may quite well be the case with those who oppose Malthus and his neo-Malthusian successors, supposing that the latter are wrong. We may proceed, therefore, on the assumption that our investigation may not be

---

[1] In its original form this essay formed part of a long and detailed paper on "The Biological Basis of Sexual Repression and its Sociological Significance," *British Journal of Psychology—Medical Section*, 1921, I, pp. 225–280), in which I tried to show that sexual repression was the psychological aspect of that antagonism between ' Individuation ' and ' Genesis ' to which Herbert Spencer had drawn attention in his *Principles of Biology*, an antagonism that was implied also in the work of Malthus on population and that of Darwin on biological evolution.

without value, even in the event that the standpoint from which it was written should turn out to be untenable.

At the risk of seeming didactic or pedantic, we shall assign numbers to the motives that we are about to pass in review, in the hope of making our exposition somewhat clearer. Two cautions, however, must be added. In the first place, there is nothing specially significant about the actual order of our exposition. Actually perhaps the most important motives, in the sense of exercising the greatest influence among the greatest number of persons, are those that we have numbered 3 and 7. In the second place, it should be remembered that in any given individual mind the motives can be present in almost any combination; even those that are logically contradictory can be simultaneously operative, owing to the peculiar stratification of the mind and its capacity for 'ambivalence' (the adoption of opposite attitudes towards a single thing or person). Our list of motives, in fact, provides us only with a general scheme which may help to disentangle the complex forces that result in hostility to birth control on the part of any given person.

II

SOME UNCONSCIOUS MOTIVES IN THE OPPONENTS OF BIRTH CONTROL

With this much said, we may proceed to our enumeration.

(1) Among the motives of a more general kind is one to which Freud has already drawn attention as playing a part in the resistance to the doctrines of Darwin, *i.e.*

the blow to human Narcissism involved in the recognition of the fact that human life is essentially of the same nature, and is subject to the same conditions, as that of the lower animals.[1] Just as it was unpleasant for man to abandom his claim to a special creation at the hands of the Divinity and to admit that he was of the same descent as his humbler brethren, so too it is unpleasant for him to realize that he is still subject to the same biological laws which control the destiny of the other animals; especially since these laws reveal the existence of an ever-present danger to human life, which it would be much more agreeable to overlook. Man is (not unreasonably) a little proud of his unique position in the world of living beings, and of the powers over the forces of Nature which he, alone of these beings, is able to wield. More particularly is he proud of his latter-day achievements in this direction, which have enabled him to modify his physical environment in a manner undreamt of by his ancestors and to gratify desires the fulfilment of which had up till comparatively recently seemed utterly impossible. It is humiliating to realize that in spite of this vast progress in the mechanical arts man is, *under actually existing conditions*, still subject to the struggle for existence in essentially the same way as are the other animals; that at the present moment there are millions who are inadequately provided with the mere necessities of life; and that, increase production and improve distribution as we may, it seems exceedingly unlikely that

[1] "A difficulty of Psycho-Analysis," *International Journal of Psycho-Analysis*, 1920, I, 17. As Freud points out, this attitude of superiority is not one that is characteristic of the primitive human mind, infantile or savage ; but it is evidently one that acquires great strength in the higher stages of culture. The study of this change in man's attitude towards the animals is an interesting chapter of psychology that has still to be written.

we could so augment the supply of necessaries as to provide a comfortable livelihood for the immensely increased numbers that would result from a full exercise of reproductive power.[1] In order to avoid the recognition of this painful fact there is a tendency to declare, first, that Malthus's principle of the pressure of population upon the means of subsistence is quite generally untrue; or, failing this, that it does not apply to present-day conditions, with the greatly increased powers of production which we now possess (ignoring the fact that the population to be fed has increased concomitantly with the increasing supply of food); or, failing this again, that, although it may apply to the economic conditions as they exist at the moment, this need give us no serious concern, since the difficulties thus arising may easily be abolished in the near future—by such measures as increased emigration, cultivation of new land, intensive agriculture or improved methods of distribution (neglecting again to take into consideration that, unless the ratio of population to subsistence be adequately controlled, any increased supply of necessaries will be spent in maintaining a larger number of inhabitants at much the same economic level as before). This last, in particular, is a very favourite method of escape from the unwelcome proposition, as any speaker who has endeavoured to discuss the law of Malthus with any kind of audience, will readily testify. There is a quite amazing unwillingness to recognize the difference

[1] Some countries have a birth-rate of 50 per thousand or more, others a death-rate of 10 per thousand or less. If these figures held of one and the same country (and under favourable conditions there is no reason why they should not), there would be an increase of 40 per thousand, or 4 per cent. per annum, which, if continued, as C. V. Drysdale pointed out a good many years ago (*The Malthusian Doctrine in its Modern Aspects*, 1917), would mean approximately a doubling of the population about every seventeen and a half years or a fifty-fold increase in a century.

between what C. V. Drysdale has aptly called static and kinetic overpopulation. Static overpopulation would exist if the earth were already peopled up to its final limit of production—a state of affairs which neither Malthus nor any other sane writer on population has ever regarded as one that need immediately concern us. What is serious is kinetic overpopulation, the fact that population tends to *increase* faster than the means of subsistence, so that at any given moment the population is likely to be greater than the available supply of necessaries. It is perfectly true that, with luck or economic progress, the supply may in another year or so be ample for the same-sized population; but this does not prevent the actual shortage now; nor does it prevent the population correspondingly increasing, so that in the given time the increased supply of necessaries will still be inadequate to meet the demand. The same applies to distribution. Scarcity in one place may, at any moment, very well coincide with glut in another, a disproportion that better methods of transport and distribution might well remedy. But this is no consolation to those who are actually suffering from the scarcity; and by the time a more efficient or equitable method of distribution has been brought into operation, human fertility may wipe out the benefits that would otherwise accrue. Only those who have endeavoured to make clear this relatively simple distinction between what *is* available and what *could be* (but is not actually) available can appreciate the intense obtuseness that is constantly displayed even by intelligent people in this matter—a matter that is, of course, of fundamental importance for an appreciation of Malthus's law of population, and one that is moreover acquiring a new and sinister significance in these days of combined scarcity and 'over-production.' This, then, we may regard as the first of the great psychological difficulties in the way of a ready acceptance of neo-Malthusianism—the blow to man's vanity involved in the recognition of the fact that, in spite of his exceptional capacity to bring about the satisfaction of his desires by the appropriate modification of his environment, he is nevertheless still subject to the law of Nature which ordains that the maximum of any given species shall be rigidly determined, not by the reproductive inclinations or capacities of that species, but by the supply of necessaries that is available for its use.

(2.) A second factor of importance—one that is in certain significant respects related to the above—consists in the unwillingness of men to abandon a certain childlike attitude in virtue of which they are prone to believe that all their needs will be provided for without the necessity for forethought or effort on their own part. Such an attitude may be fostered at a relatively conscious and superficial mental level by any social system in which the less thrifty and capable members of the community are (partially or wholly) maintained at the expense of the more able and far-seeing individuals. More fundamentally, however, the attitude is one that is adopted towards God or Nature rather than towards the community. It finds expression in such well-known phrases as "Bountiful Nature" and "Providence never sends mouths but it sends food" (statements which every serious student of biology and economics knows to be profoundly untrue in the sense that is intended), and may be regarded as a particular aspect of a more general view, according to which the welfare of men is in the hands of a beneficent deity, whose constant vigilance relieves the human race of the necessity for foresight and makes it a virtue to "take no thought for the morrow," since to do otherwise would imply distrust of, or disbelief in, the deity in question.

In the light of psycho-analysis it is easy to see that this attitude is principally derived:—(a) from the positive (or loving) elements of the parent-regarding complexes, the unlimited power and beneficence originally attributed to the parents being displaced on to the more abstract personalities of God or Nature; (b) from displaced Narcissistic tendencies which co-operate towards the same end, the omnipotence of the parent or of God being partly derived from a projection of the original (infantile) "omnipotence of thought." The concept of the monotheistic Christian God or of his more modern counterpart, Nature, is deeply imbued with this influence (the former representing—at least predominantly—a father substitute, the latter a mother substitute). Thus the so frequently expressed blind confidence in the forthcoming of adequate sustenance for human populations, no matter how fast they multiply, represents a regression to an infantile level of thought and feeling. It is clung to with all the tenacity characteristic of early fixations; any attempt to overcome this confidence and to make an unbiassed scrutiny of the actual relationship between mouths and food being opposed with an energy that derives its force from a dim realization of the fact that such a scrutiny would threaten with destruction the pious and pleasing delusions which have been built up round this subject; since it would show that the supposed guarantee of an ample supply of the necessaries of human life at the hands of a beneficent deity does not in fact exist, and that, in consequence, man is largely dependent on his own efforts for such supply of these necessaries as he may enjoy.

(3) While there are thus certain psychic mechanisms which make it difficult for us to realize that Nature herself (through her inability to provide sustenance for all who are or could be born) is in the last resort responsible for the shortage of necessaries, our past history and development have at the same time impelled us to look elsewhere for the cause of our troubles, thus adding an active factor of misconception to the passive factor of want of recognition considered under the last heading. The understanding and control of natural forces (such as are involved, for instance, in agriculture or the construction of dwellings) belong to a comparatively recent chapter of human history. Before such understanding and control had been acquired, it was useless to turn to Nature for the alleviation of distress. On the other hand, we have been accustomed all through our history (human and pre-human) to compete with other beings, belonging to our own or to some different species, for the available supply of food. The struggle for existence has indeed, in all probability, fostered this tendency, allowing those to survive who competed most successfully and eliminating those whose ability to assert themselves against competitors was insufficient. This being the case, we still tend in the face of any difficulty or disaster to turn in anger against our fellow-men rather than to seek for the explanation and correction of our troubles in terms of natural science. The arousal of individual, national, or class hatred is thus a much easier matter than the development of interest in scientific remedies for sociological or economic troubles; and the hatred thus engendered may be responsible

for lines of conduct directly opposed to the dictates of scientific economics.

In national affairs this tendency may co-operate with others (notably 5, below) in producing a fierce demand for fresh territory for the expansion of an overflowing population, to the complete neglect of the more pacific alternative of so controlling population that it can live comfortably on the land already available. The ex-Kaiser, with his customary lack of discretion, truthfully but tactlessly admitted this motive for Germany's attitude at the beginning of the Great War. Since then it has been openly admitted as a justification for aggressive acts or gestures on the part of Italy and Japan, and (since the Nazi rule) once again in Germany.

In class antagonisms this same tendency has been shown in the opposition to birth control on the part of the employing class, on the ground that it would tend to do away with the supply of cheap labour. Socialists have been even more uncompromisingly hostile in their attitude, since the neo-Malthusian doctrine seemed to indicate that the cause of poverty was to be found at least as much in the disproportionate niggardliness of nature (disproportionate, that is, to the powers of reproduction with which she has endowed her creatures) as in the acquisitiveness of the wicked capitalist, and that, as a remedy for poverty, birth control might be just as potent as the overthrow of capitalism. Indeed, there can be little doubt that socialist opposition has been one of the biggest obstacles both to the impartial theoretical evaluation of Malthus's law and to the practical spread of birth control—and this ever since Godwin's original controversy with Malthus when the latter first enunciated his law, right up to the present day, when the increasing powers of production that

science has put into man's hands has made it appear all
the more plausible that poverty is due entirely to
capitalistic oppression or mismanagement.   Such an
attitude is psychologically very comprehensible, but
yet logically quite unreasonable.   It is perfectly true
(and since the last year or two it is becoming increas-
ingly admitted) that the present capitalistic system has
shown itself quite incapable of satisfactorily exploiting
for the general welfare the scientific power over natural
resources that we actually possess, and to this extent
has a grave responsibility for the existing widespread
distress.   But it is equally true that a successful socialism
would have to control not only production and distribution but the increase of population.   No neo-
Malthusian maintains that birth control is a social
panacea; it can, however, very reasonably be maintained
that control of population is essential to the success of
any thoroughgoing scheme of social improvement
whatsoever, since without it even the greatest increase
in the necessities of life is likely to be used up in keeping
a greater number of persons at the same level as before.
It is a remarkable testimony to the general neglect of
population problems that this all-important factor in
planning should have received so little attention at the
hands of the Soviet Government in Russia.

In this general tendency to lay the blame for our
misfortunes on our fellow-men rather than on Nature,
we can once again (as in the case of 2 above) see the
operation of parental complexes.   Nature is, as before,
regarded as a beneficent mother who means well by her
children, and who would fain provide amply for their
needs.   Her kindly intentions are, however, frustrated
by the wicked interference of human enemies or
oppressors, who (it is supposed) have unjustly appro-

priated an altogether undue share of her bounty. These oppressors (the enemy nation or the enemy class) are then looked upon with feelings derived by a process of displacement from those originally directed to the hated father, who (in the early days of our family life) made unwelcome demands upon our mother's love, which we should have liked to keep entirely for ourselves. Alternatively, the feelings in question may be derived from these with which we regarded the competing claims of our brothers and sisters; though it would seem that our attitude towards these latter is often secondary to that which we have already developed in relation to our father. In this way the Œdipus Complex and its derivatives, which have their roots in the nursery, may distort the political and economic judgments of our adult years, making us blind to the existence of a biological factor, the understanding and control of which are of supreme importance for human progress.[1] It would seem powerfully to reinforce (or perhaps, more accurately speaking, to embody or provide a channel for) that natural and instinctive tendency, which our past history and evolution has probably implanted in us, to turn in fury on our fellow-men when we find ourselves frustrated, rather than to seek the cause of our unhappiness in a natural law, which must be circumvented if our troubles are to cease.

[1] The operation of the Œdipus Complex is here very similar to that in many forms of patriotism, in which, as several psycho-analytic writers have shown, our country (or ' mother-land ') is regarded as our mother, who is attacked by a wicked enemy, our father—a psychological fact which was exploited (unwittingly, perhaps, but very appropriately) in the traditional question asked of conscientious objectors in the war. The chief difference between the two cases is that in this type of patriotism it is the mother who is chiefly threatened, whereas in the attitude towards neo-Malthusianism that we have been considering we ourselves (*i.e.* her children) are regarded as the principal sufferers from our father's aggressiveness and importunity.

B

(4) While keeping thus in mind the very significant fact that the struggle for existence has implanted in us a tendency to look to our fellow-creatures rather than to Nature as the cause of any scarcity of food or other necessaries that we may experience, this must not blind us to the correlative fact that the human mind has, in the course of its evolution, also acquired a tendency to overcome the impulses which lead men to fight and compete with one another. The immense advantages of co-operation and socialization (with the moralization that these imply) are obtainable only with the help of a very considerable degree of inhibition of the more primitive egoistic trends, and, although this inhibition is phylogenetically a comparatively recent growth and therefore corresponds to the more superficial levels of the mind, its importance for our present subject is but little inferior to that of the egoistic and hostile tendencies themselves. The gregarious and social tendencies, with their resulting inhibitions embodied in that moral factor of the human mind which psycho-analysts have termed the super-ego, exercise a more or less constant repressive influence on hatred and pugnacity, and in so doing tend to repress also the memory or appreciation of situations calculated to arouse strife or hatred. It has thus come about that, along with the unwillingness to perceive private causes of hostility between definite individuals (*e.g.* between the different members of a family), men have also been loath to recognize the existence of certain general causes of hostility. Among these general causes, the scarcity of the necessaries of life, with the inevitably resulting competition for the inadequate available supply (between individuals, classes, nations, or races), is by far the most fundamental, the most widespread and the most persistent. All

those persons whose predominant mental trends are largely under the influence of a powerful inhibition of the hostile impulses—including a very large proportion of political, moral and religious reformers—have therefore been at pains to overlook the continuance of the struggle for existence among mankind; or, if they could not overlook it, to prove that it need not exist; and modern Western culture, which has so largely taken its ideals from reformers of this stamp, has for the most part followed in this respect the biassed guidance of its leaders. That Nature herself, through the disproportion between the powers of reproduction on the one hand and the available supply of nutriment on the other, is responsible for making every man to some extent the enemy of every other, is for most idealists a proposition too unpleasant to be tolerated. Hence in minds of this sort there is a potent reason for the rejection of the doctrines of Darwin, and more especially of those of Malthus (where the struggle for existence is more definitely brought into relation with mankind). The more constructive types of Socialism and Internationalism aim alike at the abolition of hostility and competition between members of the human race, and both have been in a large measure blind to the powerful obstacles which Nature has placed in the way of a realization of their ideals.[1]

In this respect the Germans again would seem to have enjoyed a less distorted vision than ourselves. Although they may not have been altogether guiltless of sometimes placing undue emphasis on just those aspects of biology which seemed best to fit their pre-conceived

---

[1] Of course I do not mean to imply these ideals are necessarily unrealizable, but only that as a condition of their realization the natural obstacles opposed to them must be faced and overcome, and not neglected.

political opinions, they were at any rate not blind to the fact that the biological laws enunciated by Darwin indicated the inevitability of the struggle for existence so long as population continued to press upon the means of subsistence—a fact which many of our own thinkers, misled by a more idealistic political philosophy, had overlooked. A sounder idealism of the future, based on knowledge rather than on neglect of unpleasant realities, may some day, we may hope, succeed in combining a genuine aspiration for the abolition of the cruelties involved in the struggle for existence with a due appreciation of the bearing of biological truths upon human social life.

Within the sphere of national, as distinct from international, politics, the same influences have clearly been at work. The supporters of the doctrines of Malthus have almost always been conservatives or individualists of the tougher sort, while to the more tender-minded among social reformers (from Godwin onwards) "hardhearted Malthusianism" has ever been repellent. To the prevailing socialistic tendencies of political thought Malthusianism is unacceptable, not only for the reasons considered under the last heading, but also because it implies a recognition of the circumstances making for hostility between man and man which the socialistic idealist is anxious to avoid. And yet it is only by taking the necessary steps towards overcoming the struggle for existence (*i.e.* by adjusting population to available subsistence) that any successful socialism would be possible.

But the doctrines of Malthus are unacceptable, not only for the reason that they draw attention to causes of hostility which, in virtue of our philanthropic tendencies, we would fain overlook. These doctrines are also unwelcome in a more positive way, inasmuch as they threaten to remove some of the means by which these tendencies are at present gratified. As a result of the development of the gregarious tendencies, charitable or kindly behaviour towards our fellow-men has come to be in some respects a source of considerable pleasure. Pleasure of this kind can be most easily and satisfactorily obtained by the direct alleviation of the sufferings of those who are less well endowed with the good things of life than we ourselves. Malthusianism, although it promises a much more thorough remedy for social and economic troubles than any of the usual charitable activities—since it deals with the cause of the troubles and not merely with their symptoms, is yet in some ways less calculated to arouse the interest and enthusiasm of the charitably disposed: (*a*) because these latter are already concentrated on their own schemes of social reform, which they are usually unwilling to abandon, (*b*) because the advocacy of Malthusianism does not involve the actual giving of anything—an element which is essential to the full gratification of our charitable tendencies, (*c*) because Malthusianism ultimately threatens to do away with poverty altogether, and thus to deprive us of the pleasures we derive from the exercise of charity (the heightening of our moral self-esteem, the sense of our own power, and superiority—involving as this does a by no means negligible element of *Schadenfreude*—the satisfaction of the displaced anal-erotic tendencies involved in giving and of the displaced parental feelings involved in protecting, etc.).

The subject of parental feelings brings us finally to one other cause of resistance to the Malthusian doctrine which can most appropriately be considered under this head. The sacrifice that parents are called upon to make on behalf of their children[1] naturally leads to some degree of resentment and hatred on the part of the parents—feelings which find their primitive expression in the widespread practice of infanticide, child sacrifice, exposure and abortion; but which, in the course of moral development, have necessarily been subjected to a very high degree of repression. Now abstention from conception is, from certain points of view, only a further stage in the series of actions involved in infanticide or abortion, and constitutes to some extent an expression of hostility to the unconceived child in the same way that abortion and infanticide constitute expressions of hostility to the child before or after birth respectively. The repression of child-hatred, which has led to the condemnation of these latter practices, has to some degree extended to the neo-Malthusian methods of contraception. Hence the tendency to look upon contraception as being (like infanticide or abortion) a kind of " murder," since all three practices gratify the same repressed (murderous) desires—a tendency that is probably to a large extent responsible for the very frequent identification of contraception with abortion and for a considerable portion of the moral indignation felt against the former practice.[2]

(5) Connected also with the impulses making for gregariousness and socialization is another factor of some importance, i.e. the tendency to feel faith and confidence in the existence or presence of large numbers of our fellow-creatures. Human history has in the main

---

[1] Cf. the present writer's *Psycho-analytic Study of the Family*.

[2] There are of course certain other important reasons for the identification in question. Cf. under 7.

favoured the creation of large communities. Wherever economic conditions have permitted of a relatively dense population and social development has proceeded far enough to permit of such a population being knit into a social whole, the larger groups have enjoyed certain advantages, such as greater power in war, greater division of labour and a more active and diversified mental life and outlook. In consequence of these advantages, they have usually proved superior to their smaller neighbours, whom they have eventually for the most part either exterminated or incorporated within themselves. The human race, having thus learnt in the course of its history, to appreciate the advantages of numbers, is apt to regard with distrust any social tendency that makes, or seems to make, for smaller populations. Actually, however, the size of groups has only been one factor in success. Especially after a certain stage of evolution has been reached, the degree of culture possessed by a community is apt to become an equally important factor, and (in accordance, the present writer would like to add, with the general Spencerian law of the antagonism between individuation and genesis) increased culture tends as a rule to go with diminished reproductivity. The older and more primitive tendency to place confidence in numbers is therefore apt to give rise to alarm at the threatened decrease in fertility that higher culture usually entails, and, since at the present moment birth control is one of the most important methods of reducing fertility, this alarm naturally attaches both to the practice of contraception and the theory of neo-Malthusianism which points to its desirability. That the faith in numbers still constitutes an influence of very genuine importance was illustrated very forcibly by our con-

fidence in the irresistible power of the "Russian steam-
roller" at the beginning of the Great War and the corresponding fear of Russia on the part of Germany—both
confidence and fear being, as it turned out, exaggerated,
in consequence of a failure to take due account of
qualitative as well as quantitative factors.   Another
illustration is afforded by France, where, in spite of a
very widespread application of neo-Malthusian principles in private life, there exists something in the nature
of a panic with regard to the low birth-rate and more or
less stationary population—a panic that is resulting in
a wild clamour for more births, without any realization
of the conditions or consequences of a higher birth-
rate.

This tendency, in so far as it is due to the action of
gregarious or social impulses, is apt to be powerfully
reinforced by a displaced self-regarding (Narcissistic)
impulse, which, through an identification of the self
with the community or state [1] to which the individual
belongs, sees in the increasing numbers of the latter
an increase in the glory or safety of the Self—and is
therefore unwilling to countenance anything that may
reduce the population of the state, since in any such
reduction it is apt to see a menace to the Ego.   This
factor is, in its turn, intimately connected with one
that we shall consider below (6b).

(6) One of the most important and direct of all the
influences opposed to the appreciation and understanding of the need for birth control is derived from
the sexual impulse itself.   By general consent this
impulse is among the strongest that we have, and, as all
control and frustration of impulse is unpleasant, there

[1] Cf. Ernest Jones, " War and Individual Psychology," *Papers on Applied
Psycho-analysis.*

is a natural temptation to ignore the existence of a situation which urgently demands the setting of limits or conditions to sexual gratification.   As already mentioned, I am not speaking so much of the practical inconvenience of certain birth control methods, irritating as these undoubtedly can be.   I am dealing here rather with the general theory of neo-Malthusianism, which stresses the necessity for the use of these methods as the only alternative to over-population or to wide-spread abstinence from " normal " sexual intercourse.

The original doctrine of Malthus himself presented the situation in a particularly disagreeable aspect, since on his view the abolition of over-population with its attendant evils of poverty, war, disease and premature death required the very extreme degree of sexual inhibition involved in the postponement of all sexual relations till relatively late in life.   According to him, humanity was in a horrible dilemma.   Birth control, at some slight sacrifice of money and convenience, gets over the difficulty so far as direct sexual pleasure is concerned.   It is an ingenious triumph over Nature and provides an escape from the dreadful alternatives to which Malthus had so eloquently drawn attention. But it leaves untouched the restraints on reproduction, as distinct from those on sexual pleasure.   Now there can be no doubt that the immediate instinctive urgency of the sexual desire relates to the sexual act (in one or other of its various possible forms) rather than to repro-duction.   How far the failure to make full use of the actual reproductive powers gives rise to dissatisfaction, to a sense of unfulfilment and frustration, is a matter on which (masked as it is by the more clamorous demand for sexual gratification) we have still comparatively little knowledge.   It may be that this failure gives rise to some obscure but deep-rooted trouble of a biological or physiological order, manifesting itself mentally in some vague anxiety or discontent. This is perhaps especially the case with women, whose physiology is more deeply and intimately affected by their reproductive functions than is that of men. But this at present is little more than a surmise. What we do know is that failure and restriction of reproduction may give rise to certain purely (or at least primarily) psychogenic troubles, troubles which in some cases may be largely a matter of individual psychology, but which in others have a social root. In so far as influences of this kind are at work in the community, it is understandable that they will cause opposition not only to Malthus's original law of population but to the neo-Malthusian method of escaping some of the undesirable consequences of this law. We cannot here attempt an enumeration or description of all the possible forms of such influences. We may, however, mention three factors with regard to which anthropological or psychological research has produced specially striking or important evidence. These may perhaps be most conveniently classed as sub-groups under the present heading.

(6a) At certain primitive levels of thought there appears to be a confusion between human fertility and the fertility of the plants and animals which serve for human food. This is shown in a very considerable number of primitive religious and social customs, underlying which are ideas to the effect that barrenness in a woman or impotence in a man may cause infertility both among men and among animals and that the fertility of plants or animals may be increased by the vigorous practice of sexual intercourse by human beings (a supposition which has encouraged the holding of sexual orgies at certain times of the year; such orgies —in actual or symbolic form—being a prominent feature of festivals of the Carnival type.)[1] It is not necessary here to enter into the psychological causes of this confusion:[2] it is sufficient to point out that this confusion must of necessity prevent a proper appreciation of the true relations between population and the means of subsistence, since it identifies the very factors which in any such appreciation must be rigorously kept apart.

It is only fair, however, to add that this factor is doubtless operative to a much greater extent among primitive communities than among modern civilized societies, although relics of its influence may perhaps still be found among the more pastoral and agricultural sections of the latter.

(6b) For a variety of reasons, into which again it is not necessary to enter here,[3] the Narcissistic tendencies find a very special degree of satisfaction in the development and exercise of the reproductive functions and a

[1] Vide e.g. Frazer, *Spirits of the Corn and the Wild*, II, 332 ff.

[2] Which are doubtless complex in nature, but in which the following four factors will probably be found to be of importance : (a) the projection of human sexual desires on to Nature, in connection with the repression of these desires, (b) the Totemic identification of animals or plants with human parents, (c) the " omnipotence of thought " manifested in the control of the food supply by homœopathic magic, (d) a " return of the repressed," in so far as the practice of this magical control furnishes an excuse for the indulgence of sexual activities which would be otherwise prohibited.

[3] They are doubtless connected in the ultimate resort with the biological conditions which make it advantageous for any race or individual to have reproductive powers and tendencies as vigorous as the economic conditions of life and the energy required for purposes of Individuation will permit (conditions which were considered in the above-mentioned paper on " The Biological Basis of Sexual Repression," *British Journal of Psychology, Medical Section*,1921, Vol. I) ; and also, more immediately, with the factors referred to under headings 1 and 5 of this paper.

corresponding dissatisfaction in anything that appears to entail a weakening or atrophy of these functions. Owing to the strength of the general sexual inhibitions in modern societies, our pride and joy in the use of the sexual organs can no longer find expression in the crude manner characteristic of the phallic cults of more primitive ages: but some remnants of our former attitude in this matter are still shown: positively, in the continued employment of phallic symbolism; negatively, in our somewhat morbid horror or disgust of anything that threatens the existence or activity of the sexual organs, *e.g.* castration or impotence. The tendencies underlying this attitude ally themselves with the motives which lead us to have confidence in a numerous population and distrust of any decrease of population or of any diminution in the rate of increase — motives which we have already studied (5 above).

That these tendencies are in reality derived from the psychic sources to which we have just referred is shown by the fact that those who extol most lavishly the benefits of a high birth-rate and who exhibit most alarm at the voluntary control of births (which they are fond of designating "race suicide") are to be found chiefly among elderly persons (whose sexual power has departed or is declining), or else among confirmed bachelors, celibate priests or unmarried women. In the case of these persons there has probably occurred a projection of the primitive pride in fertility and sexual potency, or of the fear resulting from sexual inhibitions or from impotence. The pride that would find a more primitive expression in the individual's own fertility is displaced on to the fertility of the race or community, with resulting joy in a high birth-rate and hatred of any doctrines or social movements calculated to bring about a decline in reproduction.[1]

(6c) There is also another way in which the Narcissistic tendencies co-operate with the reproductive trends to make the neo-Malthusian doctrines appear unwelcome. Among the most common and important forms of displacement of the Narcissistic elements of the Libido is the transference of love from self to offspring—an individual's children being regarded as an extension or a re-incarnation of himself. The love of our children constitutes at once a socially more permissible and a biologically more advantageous form of Narcissistic gratification than the cruder forms of conceit, self-admiration or auto-erotic satisfaction; while the continuation of our own lives through those of our children and our children's children affords us at the same time the nearest possible approach to the immortality which, in virtue of our Narcissism, we so earnestly desire. It is therefore not surprising that the displaced tendencies which have found a satisfactory substitute in this way oppose everything which threatens to rob them of this substitute. Now it can scarcely be doubted that the practice of neo-Malthusianism does bring with it a certain degree of danger to the continuance of the

[1] In actual practice this attitude is effective in preventing a proper appreciation of the Malthusian doctrine, not only by direct opposition, but—especially in so far as it works with modern statistical weapons—by fostering an undue concentration of attention on birth-rates, to the neglect of death-rates and other important factors which must be taken into account in any unbiassed consideration of the problems of population ; the subject of birth-rates being of course more in the direct line of displacement of interest in minds of the type here referred to. So great is the distortion thus introduced that the more violent type of *répopulateur* seems often to be of the opinion that population depends simply upon the birth-rate, as if such factors as death-rate, immigration and emigration did not exist !

individual family. The process of "peopling down" to a relatively high level of comfort entails—except under unusually favourable circumstances—such a limitation of the numbers of the children born to each marriage, as to expose the family to greater danger of extinction through accident or disease. This real increase of danger to the continued existence of any given family under a Malthusian régime is apt to be exaggerated in imagination: (*a*) through reinforcement by unconscious psychological factors, particularly those referred to under (6*b*); (*b*) through failure to take into account the fact that the increased danger in question is to some considerable extent counterbalanced by the fact that a decrease in the number of children per family usually brings with it a more favourable environment for each individual child, the increase of danger to the family as a whole being thus by no means directly proportional to the decrease in the number of children, as is sometimes erroneously assumed. The fear thus engendered and exaggerated is apt to exercise a very real influence in the rejection of neo-Malthusian ideas.[1]

(7) As in the case of the aggressive tendencies which are opposed to birth control, so also in the case of the

---

[1] It is interesting to note, however, that the real danger on which the fear rests (and consequently to some extent the fear itself) may be expected to diminish somewhat as the practice of neo-Malthusianism becomes more universal. At present those who do practise family limitation are forced to " people down," not only to the limit required for the preservation of their own standard of living, but to the still lower limit required for the provision of a surplus devoted to the practical maintenance of the large families of those sections of the community who produce more children than they themselves are able to provide for. In so far as the latter classes in turn adopt the practice of family limitation, the burden of providing for those who cannot support themselves or be supported by their own families will become less, with the result that (other things equal) a rather large number of children per family will become possible in the case of the upper and middle classes, upon whom this burden principally falls.

sexual tendencies, a negative as well as a positive aspect has to be distinguished. Paradoxical and illogical as it may appear, neo-Malthusianism may, as we have seen, arouse opposition both because it runs counter to certain hostile tendencies (3 above) and because it runs counter to the inhibition of hostile tendencies (4 above). In a similar way this same doctrine is unwelcome both because it threatens the active manifestations of the sexual tendencies (6 above) and because it threatens the repressions thereof. It is repellent, not only because it reveals the necessity for sexual inhibition, but also because it is too intimately concerned with sexual matters, appeals too strongly to sexual interests and desires, and appears indeed in some respects to open up greater possibilities of sexual freedom and enjoyment; so that the far-reaching and elaborate repressions that have been built up in the course of human cultural development become in their turn operative in preventing the recognition of the biological and sociological facts to which neo-Malthusianism draws attention. The objections to birth control springing from sexual inhibitions are indeed so powerful, widespread and persistent, that, as we have already indicated, they seem to share with the political objections the rather doubtful honour of being the most striking of all the psychological factors which oppose their influence to unbiassed discussion and consideration of the problems of population.

The influence of sexual repression manifests itself of course as a general deterrent to all direction of thought upon matters connected with sexual life: in this respect questions concerning population suffer no more and no less than other problems dealing with sex. But sexual repression also affects neo-Malthusianism in more specific ways. Firstly, because the consideration of birth control involves an intrusion into the intimacies of married life—a sort of reserved territory which has been left relatively free of prohibitions on condition that it is not too often or too openly discussed. Secondly, because the use of contraceptives (which have as a rule to be procured—and in some cases also adjusted—"in cold blood") implies a deliberate hope or intention of carrying out the sexual act, and is therefore apt to stir up resistances which can sometimes be evaded so long as the persons concerned can shirk the recognition of their erotic tendencies, rationalizing their behaviour until such time as sexual desire is strong enough to overcome all moral obstacles. Birth control is therefore liable to arouse greater guilt than is encountered when we allow ourselves to slip insensibly into a sexual situation. Thirdly, (and this is certainly the most important factor) because neo-Malthusianism—revealing as it does the possibility of indulging in sexual pleasure without incurring the penalty of parenthood—threatens to remove one of the most important restraining influences on sexual behaviour, and therefore arouses a more than usually vigorous activity on the part of the inhibiting forces. Hence the very widespread fear of "immorality" as a consequence of the general knowledge of contraceptive methods, the tendency to taboo these methods as degrading,[1] and the desire (manifested especially by

[1] A method frequently employed for this purpose at the present time is to identify or confuse them with the (in this and many other countries) illegal methods of producing abortion—a result probably due largely to the co-operation of other motives, particularly those enumerated under the headings (4), (6b) and (6c) ; the "murder" of the embryo in abortion or of the spermatozoon in preventive intercourse being (unconsciously or semi-consciously) regarded either as a gratification of (repressed) death wishes (4) or else as symbolical castration (6b and 6c).

the Roman Catholic Church) that marriage—and sexual intercourse in general—shall not be freed from its "natural" penalties. The widespread and powerful nature of the repressive forces here at work is illustrated not only by the spoken and written pronouncements of those numerous persons who are very seriously alarmed at the prospect of sexual pleasures being obtainable without the deterrent effect of the probable resulting conception, but also from the very remarkable, one might almost say pathological, blindness and ignorance displayed till comparatively recently (and to some extent still manifested) by large sections of our population as regards' the existence and procurability of contraceptives, many city dwellers passing almost daily before shops where these articles are sold but never realizing consciously the nature and purpose of the goods displayed or advertised.

Recent psycho-analytic research has shown that this fear of abolishing the penalty incurred by a tabooed action is only a particularly striking instance of a general psychological tendency. There exists in the human mind a tendency which has been called the "need for punishment"; in virtue of which suffering relieves the burden of guilt at the infringement of a taboo. In the absence of external misfortunes (which may sometimes be actively—though of course unconsciously—sought) an individual may inflict internal punishment on himself in the shape of a distressing neurotic symptom; and an element of this kind can be traced in many forms of nervous disorder. The presence of the external misfortune (which is unconsciously treated as a "punishment") relieves the individual of the guilty anxiety and tension which otherwise tends to produce the symptom. But this anxiety and guilt may (in virtue of the mechanisms of identification and

c

projection) apply not only to ourselves, but to others. Likewise the punishment. The individual may feel himself morally outraged and endangered, not only by his own trespasses but by those of his neighbours. Hence he demands punishment for his neighbours, as he would do for himself; except that, when it is an affair of others, the realization both of the guilt and of the punishment is apt to be more conscious and explicit than when it is a question of oneself. The infliction of pain on others may, however, serve as a sort of vicarious punishment, so that the individual is morally relieved at the sacrifice of a "scape-goat"—a motive that finds expression over a vast range of social phenomena, ranging from the treatment of schoolchildren and criminals to that of gods. In virtue of this tendency we rejoice in the punishment of the "wicked" and feel a very pleasant sense of moral superiority in the contemplation of their sufferings. Now in the case of sex, Nature herself appears to have provided certain forms of punishment, one of which is the procreation of unwanted children. Birth control threatens to do away with this particular punishment, and therefore produces a state of anxiety in those who experience a "need of punishment" (even though the punishment may be vicarious) with regard to sex.[1] The threatened

[1] Since the burden of procreation, regarded as a natural punishment, falls more heavily on woman than on man, woman is in this case peculiarly fitted to serve as a scapegoat for man's guilt. Under the formula of " the woman tempted me " man has always been ready to project his guilt on to woman and therefore also to assuage this guilt through her punishment. Hence arises a particular form of male objection to birth control as a device which enables woman to escape her proper punishment ; though, of course, a number of other forms of male hostility (including all those which aim at keeping woman " in her place "') may easily crystallize around this tendency, as we see in the combined anti-feminist and anti-birth-control propaganda in various European countries at the present day.

abolition of the external, "natural" punishment upsets the balance of their moral forces and produces a heightened inner tension. In their alarm they naturally oppose the means of abolishing the punishment; just as they will also oppose the removal of other sufferings associated with sex, *e.g.* those connected with venereal disease or unhappy marriage. In the light of these considerations, the intense hostility shown to birth control on the ground of its "immorality" need scarcely cause surprise.

III

SOME UNCONSCIOUS MOTIVES IN THE SUPPORTERS OF BIRTH CONTROL

We have now concluded our (doubtless incomplete) enumeration of psychological factors—other than purely conscious or rational ones—that tend to arouse opposition to the doctrine of neo-Malthusianism and the practice of birth control. As stated before we embarked on this undertaking, we started out on the assumption, which we did not here attempt to justify, that there were rational grounds for considering birth control to be of social benefit. Accepting this assumption, there is a natural tendency to suppose that those who advocate birth control do so on these rational grounds, and that it is therefore futile and superfluous to look in their case for unconscious and irrational motives such as those we have studied in the case of their opponents. Such an assumption, however, is totally unjustified. It is unfortunately not only possible, but even usual, to adopt a right conclusion on irrelevant or even on false grounds—"irrelevant" and "false" at least in a logical, as distinct from a psychological sense. Psychologically there is perhaps nearly always some link between the rational and the irrational or irrelevant motive. And of course the existence of a motive of the latter kind does not necessarily mean that the rational motive is inoperative; it means rather that the irrational motive provides some of the energy in virtue of which the rational motive is able to appeal and lead to action. We all of us recognize that there are many social movements and causes which appear to be desirable. Actually there are only a very few of these which rouse us to the point of giving time or money; and the fact that both our personal and our financial resources are limited seems scarcely a sufficient explanation of why we give our active support to some particular causes out of many that are (intellectually) possible. Psycho-analysis appears to show that in many cases the "appeal" of some particular cause comes from the fact that the rational motives in its favour are reinforced by more or less unconscious and irrational ones—the energy of the latter being to some extent displaced on to the former; so that the psychology of those who make "rational" decisions with regard to social problems and of those who make "irrational" ones is in many respects at bottom not so very different.[1]

If this is so, it is clearly our business here to deal with the supporters of birth control as we have dealt with their opponents, and to show what are the principal dynamic motives of a less obvious and conscious kind that have led them to approve of the contraceptive practices that others have so strongly deprecated.

. [1] This is obviously not the place in which to enter into the difficult question as to what *are* the essential psychological differences between true and false judgments upon social problems—a matter that involves the whole psychology of the " reality principle " and of error.

Fortunately our task is made easier by what we have already done, for the unconscious motives in favour of birth control are to a very large extent merely inversions of the motives against birth control that we have just now considered. Our treatment therefore may be relatively brief, and we may content ourselves (for here again we make no claim to cover the whole ground) by reconsidering these motives very shortly, in order to show how an opposite attitude may in each case lead to the support, instead of the condemnation, of birth control. For the sake of convenience we may now employ Roman numerals for our consideration of the motives which we have already dealt with and listed under corresponding Arabic figures.

(I) In the corresponding attitude (1) we encountered a Narcissistically determined insistence on a specially privileged position in the scheme of creation. Here (*i.e.* in the case of the neo-Malthusian) we find the abandonment of such a claim. The demands of Narcissism have been reduced or have found other outlets. The problem as to how this reduction or displacement is achieved is an interesting one, but unfortunately is too complex to be considered here in detail. The change of attitude in question has probably something in common with the change that makes it possible for a member of an aristocratic caste or family to become a socialist. It clearly involves: (*a*) a certain masochistic joy in the sacrifice of privilege, a masochism that may contain moral elements connected with the appeasement of unconscious guilt, (*b*) a sympathetic identification with those other lowlier beings (persons or animals, as the case may be) with whom the convert recognizes his community, (*c*) a hostility towards those who claim a special privilege, accompanied often by a fierce joy in dragging them from the insecure pedestals on which they would fain stand. This joy in degrading and shocking the pompous is a very real one to the rebel mind and has played a considerable rôle both in politics and science. In the latter field it was undoubtedly an important factor in the fight for Darwinism, as appears very clearly in the demeanour of that stalwart champion T. H. Huxley; and neo-Malthusianism is, after all, only the practical corollary of one of the main elements of Darwinism.

(II) Whereas the motive previously considered under the corresponding numeral depended on a fixation on an early stage of the parent-regarding attitude, in which parents tend to be looked upon as all-good and all-powerful, the motive that now concerns us springs from the period of disillusion that follows the painful process of becoming aware that one's own parents are subject to much the same limitations and deficiencies as other persons. The change of attitude involved is of the same nature as that which leads to the abandonment of the belief in an all-seeing and all-providing God, and a realization that man has got to provide for his own necessities as best he can in a hostile or indifferent universe—inevitably a bitter disillusion (as is shown by the numerous myths which attempt in one way or another to get over it and reinstate the omnipotent parent),[1] but one which tends, under some circumstances at any rate, to produce friendliness between man and man, since co-operation between equals seems the only way of making good the loss incurred by the withdrawal of parental or supernatural support. In this way (II) leads on to . . .

(III) Here parent-hatred, instead of being displaced

---

[1] Cp. Otto Rank. *The Myth of Birth of the Hero.*

on to another nation or another class, as in (3), is displaced on to Nature, who is conceived as having failed in her duty to her children, whereas mankind are looked upon rather as a band of brothers engaged in the common enterprise of wresting a livelihood from Nature. This attitude makes such an "unnatural" practice as birth control (which is sometimes indeed said to "cheat Nature") appear in a favourable light, whereas in the case of (2) and (3) it had seemed both an unjustifiable slight on Nature's bounty and a deceptive snare set by wicked and oppressive tyrants (father-figures) to distract attention from their own iniquity.

It is in this frank recognition of Nature's insufficiencies and in a consequent hostility of man to Nature that (III) differs from (4), which it resembles inasmuch as both involve the overcoming of hate. It differs also in the absence of "superiority feelings," which we mentioned under the heading of (4) as being operative in the philanthropic activities which birth control threatened to render unnecessary.

(IV) On the other hand (IV) *contrasts* with (4) in that, in the former, hostility of a certain kind finds a subtle though efficient outlet—namely against those potential beings who are prevented from coming into existence by the practice of birth control. The tendencies to child "murder" which were repressed in (4) are given free play in (IV), and to this extent birth control really does involve the same psychological factors as those that are operative in abortion and infanticide, except that in the two former the hostility has become refined by being directed against the unborn or unconceived—a process which enables us to look upon them as constituting a far lesser outrage on our moral feelings. Fundamentally the motives of the

birth controller only express the same tendencies which
were manifested in a cruder form by that tragic childhood figure "Father Time," in Hardy's *Jude the
Obscure*, in the fratricidal and suicidal action which he
explained—with so terrible an insight into economic
reality—as "done because we are too menny."

Judging from the experience of the present writer,
it would appear that (IV) is one of the most important
motives in the making of enthusiastic birth controllers.
Thus several of those who have played an active part
in the birth control movement are either members of
large families, the ever-increasing size of which they
have much resented in their youth, or else have suffered
from a considerable degree of jealousy and fear in
childhood lest their mother should have further children.
The persistence of such an attitude may cause birth
control to be unconsciously regarded as a means of
preventing the arrival of further brothers and sisters
which was at one time so much dreaded or resented.

(V) Contrasts with (5) in that there is an emphasis
on individual worth as against mere numbers. It is
the reaction of the aristocratic tendency against faith
in big battalions. The motto of the Malthusian League
for many years was, "Quality not Quantity," while the
Eugenics movement also upholds ideals which are
definitely opposed to a high valuation of mere fertility
as such. At the same time these tendencies may
perhaps be looked upon as a triumph of sublimation
over sex and reproduction.

(VI) These same tendencies are also intimately connected with (VI), under which heading come attitudes
opposite to those that we have dealt with under (6).
Sublimation is here looked upon as a superior substitute for sex. Man, therefore, who has the cultural

power implied by sublimation, is contrasted rather than identified with the fertility of Nature (VI*a*); the over-emphasis on the sexual functions falls away, since alternative values have been found (VI*b*); while, similarly, the individual feels strong enough to stand on the merits of his own personal achievements without requiring the vicarious immortality provided by descendants (VI*c*.)

It is obvious that changes of this kind require re-adjustments in the distribution and displacements of Narcissistic libido which are of profound importance for human civilization. In the individual they imply an ability to overcome that overestimation of sex, that identification of individual value with fertility and sexual potency, which constitutes one of the most serious difficulties in the way of sublimation; while in their social displacements, the capacity to take pride in the cultural achievements of one's nation (or other social group) rather than in its mere numbers or brute strength is an essential, or at any rate a highly significant, step towards the abolition of war.

(VII) Though the motives coming under (V) and (VI) are antagonistic to the sexual impulses (as expressed in a slightly displaced form), those coming under (VII) are, of course, as the opposites of the inhibitory factors considered under (7), favourable to those impulses (as expressed in their direct form). Indeed, it is the greater general freedom with regard to sex that has allowed birth control to emerge from the status of a tabooed to that of a respectable subject. In this general sexual emancipation, freedom of discussion has (in Great Britain at any rate) gone farther than freedom of action. Nevertheless, the greatly increased support for birth control that has been forthcoming in recent years does undoubtedly signify that there is now a widespread feeling that sexual pleasure under certain conditions is justified for its own sake, and not merely in virtue of the fact that it is associated with the reproductive function. And this dissociation of sex and reproduction is, from the sociological point of view, surely a momentous step; for once it is admitted that sexual intercourse is permissible because of the satisfaction that it gives, it is difficult to find any logical justification for confirming our approval of it to the case of marriage, which is a social institution primarily concerned with the procreation of children. The victory for birth control that seems to be in process of achievement thus represents a real blow at those social forces that make for restrictions upon sex. The weakest point in the present position is (as indicated at the beginning of this paper) that many who practise birth control, and enjoy some at any rate of the freedom it is able to bestow, do so with a guilty feeling that they are acting immorally and anti-socially. As long as this is the case, there is always the possibility of a violent reaction, the effects of which may wipe out the progress hitherto achieved. Expressed psycho-analytically, the present position represents an insecure triumph for the libidinal forces of the id, a triumph which is in harmony with the "reality principle," but one which is unstable because the unconscious forces of the super-ego have been little if at all modified in their attitude of disapproval. Under these circumstances a relatively very small change in the balance of the mental energies (produced either directly by internal causes or indirectly through some modification of the outer world) may result in a return of the repression and insistence on some form of "punishment."

Summarizing our review of the more unconscious and irrational forces working in favour of birth control, we can discern that they have certain tendencies in common. They all seem to involve some revolt on the part of the individual ego against the forces representing the parents, the family and the super-ego. Neo-Malthusianism seems to stand, above all, for the value of the individual and the justifiability of his desires, as against the more impersonal forces that make for the sacrifice of the individual in favour of the race, duty or tradition. As such, it seems to be in the line of progress as indicated by the aim of psychoanalytic treatment, which, according to recent formulations, is directed to the task of strengthening the conscious ego. If it is permissible to make inferences from individual psycho-therapy to the problems of social hygiene, we may perhaps be comforted in finding what thus appears to be some confirmation of our original assumption that neo-Malthusianism is socially a sound procedure. This, however, is not our main task here, which has been confined to the description of some of the unconscious factors which make objective judgment difficult in the case of birth control—as in that of so many other social matters. And we may be assured that in the long-run the scientific analysis of unconscious bias will make us more capable of taking an impartial view; in this lies perhaps the main contribution of the psychologist to the many problems that at present so urgently beset humanity.

SEXUAL AND SOCIAL SENTIMENTS[1]

I

THE ANTAGONISM BETWEEN SEXUAL AND SOCIAL SENTIMENTS

MERE superficial observation is sufficient to show that there exists a certain clash of interest between the sexual and the social sides of life. A man who falls in love tends to lose some or all of the sentiments that he has in common with his fellows and that bind him to them in a common social life. He becomes less obviously gregarious, avoids crowded places, neglects the company of his friends and may even (though this is less inevitable) become indifferent to

[1] From *The British Journal of Medical Psychology*, Vol. VII, Part II, 1927.

the desires and interests which he shares with these
friends, the interests connected with his professional,
social, political and recreative activities. On the other
hand, he acquires a new and absorbing preoccupation
in which others do not share. A formal betrothal
makes matters no better in this respect, and marriage,
though to some extent it paves the way to a fresh
equilibrium, opens up a long vista of domestic responsi-
bilities, all calculated to diminish the time and energy
for interest and activities of a more social nature.
Under these circumstances it would be quite comprehensible if the surviving members of some bachelor
circle, seeing their ranks continuously depleted by
those who have succumbed to matrimony, were to
repeat Maxim de Traille's words, " C'est désespérant,
nous nous marions tous"; words of which Stevenson
reminds us in his eloquent treatment of this very
theme in the opening pages of *Virginibus Puerisque*.
The phrase, "égoïsme à deux," so often applied to
lovers, who, in their mutual preoccupation, are forgetful
of the claims of others, adequately emphasizes also the
irritation that may be caused by the relatively asocial
character of sexual love.

Our great social institutions, our schools and colleges,
our clubs, our armies and our churches, are all concerned in some degree or other to keep sex at a distance.
Religion, always a great social force and in Christianity
one of the greatest socializing tendencies that the
world has ever known, has usually seen in sex a disruptive influence and has endeavoured as far as possible
to substitute an altruistic love of God and of our
fellow-men in which the sex passions shall as far as
possible be absent; while political movements which
have emphasized the need of love of man for man, if

less hostile to all manifestations of sex (since they lack the ascetic trend so prominent in most religions) are at any rate opposed to the more permanent and absorbing sex relations of a monogamic character.[1]

The purpose of the present paper is to inquire into the psychological and sociological bases of this antagonism.

Before we embark on this task, however, it may be well to say a word about the meaning of the terms "sexual" and "social" as they will be used here, although any definitions of this kind can only be of the most provisional and tentative character, since any attempt at more precise formulation would at once land us in difficult problems of a highly controversial nature. By "sexual" (as applied to psychological material) we mean those mental processes which tend specifically to lead up to, and (ultimately) to accompany, the reproductive act or such substitutive acts as may give gratification of a kind that is usually associated with this act. Though narrower than the meaning usually given to "sexual" by psycho-analytic writers, such a view of the sexual still has a wide range, including the phenomena of courtship and romantic love upon the one hand and auto-erotism and the perversions on the other. Accepting this, we may then go on to designate as "social" the mental processes, other than sexual, which tend to foster and accompany harmonious co-operation between the individuals of groups other than those directly determined by family relationship. The "social" in this sense obviously covers a wide field. It embraces for instance that need for, and pleasure in, the presence of our fellows,

[1] As regards Christianity, Bernard Shaw has admirably treated this matter in his Preface to *Androcles and the Lion*.

together with the sensitivity to their opinion, which has been so largely emphasized by writers on Social Psychology. But it also includes conceptual factors, such as love for and pride in a social group as distinct from the individuals composing it—factors which, as has often been pointed out, are of the very first importance for the higher forms of social conduct.

II

THE INSTINCTUAL FORCES INVOLVED
IN THIS ANTAGONISM

A thoroughgoing psychological examination of the antagonism here in question would involve an exact determination of the sources of the conative (instinctual) energy engaged in the struggle upon either side. In the present vast uncertainty concerning the nature and interrelations of the instinctual energies, any such precise determination is of course impossible. There would appear, however, to be two main trends of thought upon the matter. On the one hand are a group of well-known writers who hold that at least two independent instincts are involved, who believe that the "gregarious" or the "herd" instinct represents a source of energy (or at any rate a channel) that is quite distinct from that other source (or channel) of energy connected with the sexual instinct. Among such writers are McDougall, Trotter and MacCurdy. As regards the elements of affection involved in the more emotional or more intimate social relationships, McDougall would doubtless recognize the operation of a third instinct—the parental instinct with its correlative "tender emotion," an instinct which would here act in alliance with the herd instinct. This is perhaps the plainer and more common-sense point of view and seems (superficially at any rate) to derive some support from the behaviour of gregarious animals other than man, with whom the herd instinct may be strongly operative (perhaps most strongly operative) at those periods when sexual excitement may appear to be entirely absent.[1]

But a closer study of social behaviour and emotions shows that in many cases sexual factors may manifestly play a part in social situations, as in the promiscuous sexual gratifications of the ball-room, the sexual pre-occupations of the *flâneur* and *boulevardier*, the "smutty" stories of the smoke-room and the scandal-mongering of the drawing-room, not to speak of the less super-ficially striking but more permanently operative homo-sexual tendencies which seem usually to be discoverable where large bodies of the same sex are housed together for long periods.

Such cases, where social motives appear delicately interwoven with sexual motives, seem perhaps more in harmony with the second of the two main trends of thought referred to. According to this view, sexual behaviour and social behaviour do not spring from separate sources of instinctual energy, but represent,

---

[1] Though in domesticated gregarious animals, who have lost their sexual periodicity, there may on the contrary be an intimate mingling of sexual and social behaviour. Thus that very "ritual of recognition," with regard to which Trotter draws such a suggestive parallel between human conversa-tional openings and the (osphresiolagnic) greetings of the dog (*Instincts of the Herd in Peace and War*, p. 120), may in the latter animal very easily and rapidly lead up to behaviour of a definitely sexual kind. The dog is indeed very markedly a "polymorphous pervert," and in view of the many undoubted instinctual similarities between the human and the canine mind, its sexual and social conduct would surely well repay a more detailed and systematic observation than has yet been carried out by animal psychologists.

rather, alternative manifestations of one and the same fund of energy. The most eminent supporter of this view is, of course, Freud, in whose later works, especially in *Group Psychology and Analysis of the Ego*, the concept of the libido—already a very wide one—has been explicitly extended to cover those forms of feeling and behaviour which were regarded by the above-named authors as due to the operation of the "herd" or the "gregarious" instinct. Some of Freud's followers have pointed out that the libido theory presents—especially in its social applications—some remarkable similarities to Plato's concept of Eros, which undoubtedly covered both sexual and social forms of love. A very similar, and in some ways more illuminating, correspondence would seem to exist between Freud's use of the term libido and the Christian use of the term "love"; which, in its application both to the Deity and to our fellow-men, often carries an unmistakable erotic element,[1] an element that has been very clearly brought to light in the psychological studies of religion. In England this unitary view of the sexual and social tendencies has been supported, quite independently of Freud, in a short but striking paper by Mr Laurence Housman,[2] who, however, is more concerned with "tender emotion" than with "herd instinct," and who regards the interconnection of sexual and social behaviour to have come about as the result of a fusion of originally distinct tendencies rather than as representing the co-operation of somewhat differentiated expressions of a single original tendency. In addition to the

---

[1] Many of the hymns in present use in the English Church could, with a minimum of alteration, serve as (sexual) love songs.

[2] "The Relation of Fellow-Feeling to Sex." Publication No. 4 of *The British Society for the Study of Sex Psychology*.

D

general arguments in favour of the libido theory, Freud[1] brings forward two specific objections to the assumption of a separate and independent herd instinct:

(1) That nothing in the nature of such an instinct can be present during the early life of young children, since the child, so far from being pleased by the approach of any haphazard member of the herd, is only frightened when he sees a stranger;

(2) That, when the manifestations in question do appear, they can be shown to be in the nature of a reaction-formation to the more primitive attitude of jealousy—a reaction - formation in which a common love of the parent (or parent *imago*) plays the chief part and which results in an identification of children with one another on the basis of this common love.

This theory may perhaps appear both more complicated and more uncomplimentary to human nature than the opposite one (though the comments of those psychologists who have upheld the "herd instinct" are often far from flattering). It is a theory which (like most other theories of Freud) has been sharply criticized. I have no intention here to review the arguments in favour or against it; such a review would probably necessitate a consideration of the whole libido concept, itself a very formidable task. I only wish to emphasize that Freud's general extension of the libido concept to social phenomena has proved an extremely helpful method of approach to our especial problem of the interaction between sexual and social tendencies. I shall proceed therefore to make use for our present purpose of certain, as it seems to me, very illuminating considerations brought forward by Freud in the course of his exposition.

[1] *Group Psychology*, p. 86.

III

NATURE OF THE PSYCHOLOGICAL DIFFERENCES BETWEEN SEXUAL AND SOCIAL RELATIONSHIPS

A comparison of sexual relationships with social relationships reveals a number of important points in which they differ psychologically from each other. Among these points we may, following for the most part the lead of Freud, single out four of particular significance.

(1) The sensual element, which according to all authorities forms the nucleus of sexual passion, appears to be absent in those ties and affections which can be classed as social. In McDougall's view this implies that in these latter relationships the sexual instinct is absent, its place being taken by the gregarious instinct. In Freud's view it is the sexual instinct that is operative, but in an "aim inhibited" form, owing to the repression of the sensual elements. This process of "aim inhibition" undoubtedly constitutes one of the chief difficulties of Freud's theory, since the specific agencies at work in producing the inhibitions are at present inadequately explained; though on Freud's theory itself this is not so very astonishing, since according to this theory the "aim inhibition" in question is closely connected with those long-established and fundamental repressions that produced the "latent sexual period" at an early age in life.[1] According to Freud there is a very intimate relationship between the origin of group ties and the occurrence of this process of "aim inhibition." As regards the individual, he holds that the dissociation of the "sensual" from

[1] *Group Psychology*, pp. 72, 78.

the "tender" elements of affection, that originally takes place at the beginning of the latency period (and in reference to the parents), paves the way for all subsequent separate manifestations of the two, including the relative exclusion of the sensual elements in cases of romantic love, in friendship and in the bonds of social life; while (becoming more speculative) he assumes that in the history of the race, it was the father of the primal horde who, by his insistence on exclusive possession of the women, compelled his sons to curb their desires, thereby also enabling them to form social ties between one another.

(2) The fact that aim inhibition leads to the formation of social ties is, according to Freud, very largely due to a special characteristic of the aim-inhibited manifestations of the sexual instinct, namely their greater constancy and permanence as compared with sexual manifestations that are uninhibited in their aim; their greater permanence being itself connected with the absence of a means for the reduction of instinctual tension, such as is afforded by orgasm.

Whether or not we accept Freud's view of its causation, we must agree that this relative permanence and lack of periodicity is an important point distinguishing the social from the sexual trends, though in this respect the former have something in common with romantic love, which also has the element of permanence and which also depends, in some degree at any rate, upon an inhibition of the more sensual elements of the sex instinct.

(3) In social ties an important part is played by the process of identification—a process which, though not always absent in sexual affection (especially in sexual ties of a permanent nature), is at any rate a less essential

element in the total relationship. In a sexual relationship we desire, as Freud tersely puts it, "to have" the loved object, whereas in the more social relationships of an identificatory character, we desire "to be" those whom we admire or those with whom we have some important interest or character in common. The exact way in which this process of identification takes place is not yet clear in all respects. No doubt McDougall's "primitive passive sympathy"—a tendency in virtue of which the signs of any emotion in one individual tend directly to induce a similar emotion in another—is important here. But in any given case of identification, there are usually more complex and specific factors also at work, as a result of which the identification acquires its permanency and stability. Two factors to which Freud attaches importance in connection with the social aspects of identification are, in the first place, the necessity for a common renunciation or inhibition of love, as when children in the nursery, failing to obtain the exclusive love of their parents, come to demand, instead, equal treatment for all—the group spirit springing thus as a reaction-formation from what was originally jealousy or envy; in the second place, the identification that arises through the common substitution of one and the same object for the ego ideal of the various members of the group— as in the case of an army, the Commander of which constitutes in some sense the embodiment of the ideal of every one of his subordinates (though this relationship also has its deepest roots within the family circle). In this latter case each individual is similar to the others in what he would (in the widest sense) *like to be*; in the former case each individual is similar to the others in what he *is*. In both cases there arises the close identification of feelings and interests which is essential in a firmly knit and homogeneous group.

(4) In the fourth place it is clear that the social ties differ from sexual ties in their greater diffuseness, in the fact that there occurs a love for, and an identification with, many individuals, in the place of the concentration (for a time at any rate) of interest and affection upon a single individual, that is such a striking characteristic of sexual love. It is just in this matter of diffuseness that is to be found to a large extent the root of those typical forms of the antagonism between sexual and social interests to which we drew attention in our opening section. The concentration demanded by sexual love (especially sexual love in accordance with monogamous traditions) is undoubtedly in some important respects detrimental to the wider interests of the social life, while the claims of social life in turn make it difficult to accord that full devotion to a single individual, which the psychological process of "falling in love," and the sociological institution of marriage, so urgently demand. Successful social ties, so far as they relate to individuals, are in the majority of cases extensive rather than intensive. In so far as a social feeling can find adequate expression in a unitary sentiment, this sentiment is of a conceptual order, the love of a school, of a party, of a country, or of mankind, rather than the love of a concrete individual. The love of an individual must necessarily be of a relatively fleeting, superficial, easily replaceable kind, on pain of losing its "social" features and developing into that more private, secretive and absorbing affection which is characteristic of sexual love. It is, then, in this element of diffuseness that social sentiments differ most markedly from those formed under the impetus

of sex. The three previous features that we have referred to in this section, aim inhibition, permanence and identification are all (especially the first two) found to some extent in romantic love and in the sentiments formed between the partners of successful marriage. Aim inhibition (though not necessarily permanent) is also involved in that condition which, as Freud has endeavoured to show, possesses certain of the characteristics of "being in love"—*i.e.* hypnosis. Both romantic love and hypnosis, however, differ markedly from social ties in that they essentially involve a concentration of interest on a single individual rather than diffusion of it on a group.

IV

"HOMOSOCIALITY" AND "HETEROSOCIALITY"

With these considerations in mind, let us now turn to examine two special spheres which would seem to have a particularly important bearing upon the general problem of the antagonism between sex and society, the spheres constituted by the nexus of homosexual relationships upon the one hand and the nexus of family relationships upon the other. As regards the former (with which we will deal first, reserving consideration of the latter for Sections IX and X) we may perhaps be allowed to coin the word "homosocial" to designate "social" relationships between members of the same sex and the word "heterosocial" to designate "social" relationships between members of the opposite sex, the pair of terms being used in an analogous sense to the well-known existing pair of "homosexual" and "heterosexual," and the words "social" and "sexual" bearing the same meaning that we gave to them in Section I.

Now it would appear from common observation that the maintenance of relations upon a social rather than upon a sexual basis is much easier in the case of homosocial than in the case of heterosocial ties, and a little further consideration shows that, of the four factors enumerated in the previous section as conducing to "social" rather than "sexual" feeling and behaviour, each one is more likely to be present in a higher degree in homosocial than in heterosocial relationships.

(1) This is particularly obvious in the case of the *absence of the sensual element* of sex—"aim inhibition," in terms of Freud's view. The occurrence of homosocial feelings and practices on a definitely sensual level proves, however, that the participation of sensual elements is by no means necessarily and inevitably excluded, and the reason for their practical exclusion from the vast majority of homosocial relationships is, it must be admitted, not as yet entirely clear; this being one of those matters which, like gravitation or obliviscence, we take so much for granted that we seldom pause to ask how the usual course of events to which we are so well accustomed is actually brought about. It is a matter however which we cannot pursue in detail here. We can only note in passing:

(*a*) The biological absurdity of homosexuality (which would ensure the rapid extinction of those races or families in which the homosexual inclinations definitely preponderated over the heterosexual).

(*b*) The probable innate psycho-physiological basis of heterosexuality; this depending perhaps to some extent upon the physiological effects of internal secretions—a factor which in itself presents a great number of complex but highly interesting problems, on most of which our knowledge is still lamentably scanty.

(c) Turning to environmental influences, each individual is probably confirmed in (perhaps even guided into) a heterosexual path by the selective influence of other (heterosexual) individuals, since, in virtue of their heterosexuality, he receives greater (and less "aim-inhibited") manifestations of affection from those of the opposite sex than from those of his own sex. Psycho-analysis has made it appear probable that this selective influence may begin to operate at an extremely early age, through the heterosexual inclinations of the parents, the father tending to lavish greater affection upon his daughters and the mother upon her sons.

(d) But if the environment is in this way favourable to the development of heterosexuality, it is of course to an even greater extent unfavourable to homosexuality, through the severe social taboos attaching to the latter; though it is true that for the most part these only begin to operate at a relatively late age. It is only fair to remember also that the general taboos on sex activities as a whole may, by producing a violent inhibition of early-formed heterosexual tendencies, lead to the substitution of homosexual for the original heterosexual inclinations. (Psycho-analysis has again shown that this may take place at a very early age in reference to the Oedipus Complex.)

There can be little doubt that the predominantly heterosexual direction of the sensual elements of love brought about by these and other causes exerts a strong positive influence upon the development of homosociality. Owing to the very sureness and deep-seatedness of the inhibitions affecting active homosexuality, homosociality is apt to be freer up to a certain point than heterosociality, because there is less fear of the irruption of sexuality and the consequent conversion of social into sexual relationships. It is as though the unthinkableness of the extremer forms of bodily intimacy and sensual feeling diminish the resistances to the more superficial degrees of intimacy and feeling, such as are involved in the typical social relations; just as (to use a crude analogy) a car provided with powerful and reliable brakes, can, under ordinary circumstances, safely be driven at a much greater speed than one the brakes of which are unreliable and inefficient. Homosocial relations, though in the majority of cases they involve an almost complete renunciation of sexuality, yet offer compensations in social forms of enjoyment that are sociologically more unfettered and psychologically less inhibited than anything that is possible in heterosocial relations, where, owing to the easier transition from sociality to sexuality, the fear of such transition is ever near the surface, and has to be constantly guarded against in ways that are apt to impose severe restrictions upon the efficiency and enjoyability of social intercourse. This is a matter to which we shall return a little later.

(2) Turning now to the second of the four abovementioned factors that operate in favour of social as against sexual feeling, homosocial relations in many cases tend to enjoy a greater *persistence* than heterosocial relations in virtue of the same fact that we have just been considering, namely, the freedom of the former from the irruption of sexual tendencies. This greater freedom tends to give the homosocial relations a greater stability. In so far as we believe with Freud that sexual trends underlie social tendencies, we must

also add to this the influence of the greater steadiness and continuity of libido occasioned by the relative lack of direct sexual satisfaction. It should be noted, however, that both these greater advantages on the score of persistence are only secondary, depending as they do on the actual efficient maintenance of sexual inhibition. In so far as this inhibition is liable to break down even in homosocial relationships, these will probably enjoy no greater freedom, and therefore also no greater consequent stability, than do hetero-social relationships; while in so far as the inhibition actually does break down, the superior continuity due to sexual abstinence will also probably be sacrificed.[1] Furthermore, in so far as sexual abstinence is success-fully maintained in heterosocial relations, this advantage of homosociality is of course also lost.[2]

(3) Of the four factors referred to, the one that works most preponderantly of all in favour of homo-sociality is that of *identification*. Common sense and common observation seem both to show that one can identify oneself more easily with a person of one's own sex than with a person of the opposite sex, and the deeper studies of psycho-analysis have amply vindicated this view. Freud in his work on Group Psychology [3] enumerates three types of identification: (*a*) with an admired person, (*b*) with a person whose place it is

---

[1] In spite of this, however, Freud says (*Group Psychology*, p. 123) that " it seems certain that homosexual love is far more compatible with group ties, even when it takes the shape of uninhibited tendencies." He does not however give his reasons, only remarking that " an explanation (of this) might carry us far."

[2] The fact that in a monogamous society what is perhaps the most constant relationship of all—that of the marriage tie—is a heterosexual one, does not concern us here, since by definition we have expressly excluded family relationships from the field of the " social."

[3] *Group Psychology*, pp. 60 ff.

desired to take, (c) with a person with whom one has an emotional tie in common. Identification with some-one of the same sex is, as a rule, easier as regards all these types.

Especially important from this point of view is the third type. The nature of the emotional tie involved may of course be very varied. Freud in his support of the Darwin-Atkinson theory of the origin of society has especially emphasized the social importance of the common love, hatred, and jealousy of the brothers for the "primal father." A similar process of identification based on common emotions and sentiments of great intensity doubtless takes place to some extent in every army during war. But among the most important of such common emotional ties are probably the various sentiments connected with work. Most forms of work (especially in more primitive societies and more primitive states of culture) involve sex segregation. Men and women work at different jobs and acquire different common sentiments connected with these jobs. In virtue of the common interests thus formed they learn to identify themselves with other members of their own sex in a way that is difficult or impossible between members of the opposite sex.

(4) This leads to the last of the four factors mentioned. Many forms of work—especially men's work—(e.g. hunting and war) involve co-operation with several or even many individuals of the same sex. The social sentiments thus formed in common, tend to produce a *dispersion of the individual's love and interest* that contrasts very strikingly with the concentration of interest and affection which is characteristic of sexual relationships. Sexual intercourse, and the preliminaries that lead up to it, are to a large extent essentially and

inevitably *une affaire à deux*. Attempts to introduce third parties into sexual relationships are seldom made, are still less often successful, and always appear as something in the nature of perversions. The rise of romantic love with idealization of a single individual and the institution of monogamy, involving permanent attachment to a single individual, only serve to increase this contrast. For this reason an absorbing love or a successful marriage is in some respects a much more serious impediment to social activities than are loves of a fleeting and more sensual nature. Hence, as Shaw[1] has eloquently pointed out, it is just the happy marriages which are apt to prove most disastrous to the wider social interests. And, conversely, as Freud has shown, it is only in their cruder and more sensual forms, with exclusion of tenderness and romance, that the sexual interests can themselves be socialized and be gratified in combination with the social tendencies, as in the sexual orgy.[2]

V

THE PREDOMINANCE OF MALE HOMOSOCIALITY

Hitherto we have treated homosociality in general and have refrained from dealing—except quite incidentally—with any differences between the homosociality of the two sexes. There can be little doubt, however, that such differences exist and are important. So far as I am aware, all the authors who have approached this subject have been impressed with the greater sociality of men as compared with that of women Among anthropological writers Schurtz in particular[3]

---

[1] *Loc. cit.*   [2] *Op. cit.* p. 121.
[3] *Altersklassen und Männerbünde.*

has maintained that among many primitive peoples such male homosocial institutions as the Men's House and the Age Classes are the real carriers of culture. It is they which foster social feeling and co-operation and which provide the possibilities of social advance. In such societies, as in ours, marriage is an institution that is in many ways antagonistic to social life, this latter depending largely on the activities of young un-married men. The sexual life of these societies of young men living together is usually free and promis-cuous, contrasting strongly with the much more stable sexual connections formed later on in marriage—thus again exhibiting the fact that sexual relations of a superficial and fleeting character are in certain im-portant respects less antagonistic to social life than those of a more permanent nature. Dealing with modern civilized conditions and approaching the matter from the psychological point of view, Blüher[1] has studied some typical forms of association between boys and young men, more or less clearly based on an undercurrent of homosexuality, and he has shown the high degree of social co-operation and social feeling developed in such associations.

The club-life developed in our own country during the last century illustrates clearly both the antagonism between sexual and social sentiments and the greater development of social life among men. Until quite recently at any rate, nearly all successful clubs were confined to one sex, the other sex being for the most part rigorously excluded. Men's clubs, however, vastly predominated, both in number and in social importance, and usually exhibited a distinctly anti-feminine bias, manifesting at once a fear and a con-

[1] *Vom Gemeinschaftsleben der Jugend.*

tempt of women. The fear component of this attitude is pretty clearly due for the most part to the dread of the socially disturbing and disrupting influence of sex attraction, though it is possible that psycho-analysis might reveal the existence of more subtle and complicated motives also. The element of contempt is almost certainly dependent ultimately upon deep-seated factors, such as those based on the castration complex (contempt for women as not possessing the penis) and what might be termed the "prostitute complex" (dissociation of the elements of tenderness and sensuality, with contempt for the object that excites this latter).[1]

Among primitive peoples secret societies are undoubtedly also in many cases an important element in social life. These too are nearly always confined to one sex and generally confined to men. The same statement holds good of the analogues of these societies among civilized nations, from the very large, widespread and permanent groups, such as that of the Freemasons, to the smallest secret group in a college or a school. Such secret societies, in whatsoever stage of culture they be found, usually have as an interesting feature some form of initiation test or initiation ceremony, through which novices have to pass before being admitted to the full privileges of membership. Reik, in his penetrating psycho-analytic study of these initiation ceremonies,[2] has shown that their main purpose (for their total psychological significance is markedly complex and ambivalent) is an attempt to cement the social bonds between men (especially between the elders and the youths) by a reconciliation based on mutual sacrifice of heterosexual desires and

[1] Cf. Freud, *Collected Papers*, iv, p. 203.
[2] *Probleme der Religionspsychologie*, pp. 59 ff.

privileges—a conclusion that is in full accord with our present point of view.

VI

THE CAUSE OF THIS PREDOMINANCE

This fact (assuming it to be a fact) of the much more widespread occurrence and much greater cultural influence of associations between men as compared with those between women is obviously a matter of much interest both to the psychologist and the sociologist and we may well devote a little consideration here to its probable causes. These causes are themselves, in all likelihood, both psychological and sociological in nature. Dealing first with those in which the psychological influences appear to predominate, we may note the following:

(1) The greater Narcissism of women probably affects their social relations, as it does their directly sexual relations, by making them in certain ways more self-centred and less actively influential in their dealings with others. As in love, so also in social relations, they seek to attract others, so as to make others do things to them or for them, rather than themselves to do things to others. In a society composed exclusively of women this would tend to a less active intercourse and a consequent lesser formation of social bonds as compared with the state of affairs in a society of men, the individual members of which would exercise a more direct and active influence upon one another.

We should, however, be on guard against an over-emphasis of this factor, since some of the male substitutes for female Narcissism (*e.g.* pride in muscular development) may[1] lead to forms of rivalry which are as disrupting to social bonds as is the more passive love of the female for her own bodily beauty. Moreover it seems quite probable that the difference between the sexes that is here in question is not so strongly marked in primitive cultures as in civilized and sophisticated conditions, where women have more leisure, and also that it was not so great formerly as it is to-day. Certain changes that have taken place during the last hundred years or so point to a remarkable repression of Narcissism among men—a repression that has at any rate not taken place to a corresponding extent among women. Modern clothing, for instance, allows few outlets for personal vanity among men; to be dressed "correctly" or in "good taste" is the utmost that a modern man can hope for; all originality or beauty in clothing (to say nothing of the even more direct gratification of Narcissism in actual bodily exposure) being reserved for women. Up till recently in human history, men were dressed as gaudily and were allowed as much individuality in clothing as were women, and among primitive peoples it seems to be the men rather than the women who have leisure and opportunity for personal adornment. Such adornment, moreover, is not infrequently connected with the activities of exclusively male (secret) societies; a fact which should warn us again not to attribute too great importance to this factor of Narcissism at all times and places.[2]

(2) In the associations of women with one another there is apt to be a less sharp demarcation between

---

[1] But need not necessarily.

[2] For a fuller study of the social influence of clothing, see the present author's *Psychology of Clothes*.

E

social and sexual manifestations. In this country, for instance, terms of endearment and bodily demonstrations of affection (*e.g.* the kiss), that would be looked upon with disapproval as between men, are common enough and pass without censure in the social relationships of women. In terms of Freud's theory, in feminine homosocial relations the libido is less "aim-inhibited" than in male homosocial relations, so that there is a greater element of sensuality in the former than in the latter. But just this factor of aim inhibition we have seen to be in all probability an important condition of the development of social feelings—one of those factors that makes homosociality easier than heterosociality. So that the greater sensual gratification that women obtain from their homosocial relationships tends probably to diminish to some extent the social value of these relationships. This diminution probably works through a lessening of diffusion (the fourth of the factors mentioned in Section III) rather than a lessening of permanence (the second of the above-mentioned factors). The degree and kind of sensory stimulation in question will not usually produce such marked fluctuations of attitude as are connected with directly genital gratification, but gratification of any kind that depends partly upon bodily contacts will almost necessarily be somewhat restricted in its aim, so that at any given moment it relates to one individual, or at any rate to a very small group of individuals, rather than to the larger group of individuals in which the really social tendencies can find gratification.

Moreover, the relatively wide spread of erotic sensibility throughout the body in the case of women, as compared with the relatively concentrated erotism of men, enables women to obtain more gratification from such sexual manifestations as are admitted in female homosociality than men would from these same sexual manifestations; a circumstance that renders these manifestations less aim-inhibited (and therefore in a sense also more anti-social) than, judged by male standards, they might at first appear to be.

This feature of the erotic sensibility of women, while it thus increases the possibilities of subtle forms of sexual gratification, tends at the same time to decrease certain aspects of sexual inhibition, for (*a*) it tends to make the transition from social to (homo-) sexual modes of behaviour less clearly marked and therefore less easily guarded against, (*b*) it diminishes the danger of a rapid and abrupt transition from fore-pleasure to end-pleasure. It is this last form of pleasure—dependent as it is in normal cases upon direct stimulation of the genital organs—that usually bears the brunt of the sexual inhibitions. For this reason the non-genital activities producing fore-pleasure are apt to appear more harmless and are allowed a greater indulgence in women than in men.

By their constitution, therefore, women are thus more liable to introduce (non-genital) sexual elements into their homosocial relationships and to derive a greater satisfaction from these elements when introduced—both of these factors being antagonistic in some degree to the formation of diffused and elaborate homosocial sentiments.

(3) After this somewhat laboured argument in favour of the operation of factors which are certainly complex and, as some readers will perhaps think, extremely doubtful, it is a relief to turn to other factors, the influence of which is much less obscure and which are

more in harmony with our everyday psychological and sociological conceptions.

Among those who have made special studies of the psychology of sex there is a widely held opinion[1] that women are more monogamously and less promiscuously inclined than men—a condition that probably depends upon a lesser liability to dissociation of the sensual and the tender elements in love[2] and perhaps also in many cases upon more specific factors, such as those which Freud has suggested as connected with the loss of virginity.[3] Such greater tendency to concentrate sexual desire upon a single individual of the opposite sex undoubtedly exerts in several ways an anti-social influence. It tends to foster preoccupation with a single individual; preoccupation of a kind that renders intercourse with larger groups unnecessary and distasteful. In short it makes for permanent monogamous marriage, whereas, as we have seen, club life and social groups among those of the same sex usually fit in best with (indeed among primitive peoples often seem to imply as a necessary condition) the existence of sexual relations of a more fleeting and promiscuous kind.

It is however not only in a direct and positive way, by the withdrawal of the relatively dispersed social interests, that monogamous tendencies are hostile in homosociality. They are at least equally detrimental in another more indirect way, namely by affording

---

[1] The author would like to stress the fact that this is still really an *opinion* which has not yet been conclusively proved. It is almost certainly not true of all individuals, and here—as in other cases of sex differences—it is an extremely difficult matter to distinguish constitutional factors from the effects of sociological influences. See (4) below.

[2] Cp. Freud, *Collected Papers, loc. cit,*

[3] *Collected Papers,* iv, 217 ff,

conditions which are very favourable to the arousal of jealousy. The few following considerations should make this clear. If a man's[1] sexual love is entirely and intensely concentrated upon one woman, it is almost impossible for him to avoid some jealous suspicion of all men who approach her; such an avoidance of jealousy being only achieved in virtue of a trust in the faithfulness of the woman and in the willingness of his male companions to recognize his own exclusive rights over this woman. Unless he is very sure on these points, the canker of jealousy is very liable to disturb his relations to his fellow-men and render the finer fruits of homosocial life impossible. Certain cultures have succeeded in combating this difficulty to some extent by a more or less rigorous seclusion of women from social life altogether, as with the ancient Greeks, where, significantly enough from our present point of view, only women of promiscuous tendencies contributed anything to social culture, thus again illustrating the inverse relation between monogamy and sociality. It is only fair to note however that, as regards jealousy, the principal cause is obviously the desire for exclusive possession rather than the desire to possess one object and that the former desire may of course co-exist with polygamous tendencies or institutions, as in many eastern cultures. In modern western cultures, however, jealousy naturally most often shows itself in combination with intense desire for one object, so that monogamy and the anti - social influences due to jealousy are usually found together.

What we have said about men probably holds true,

---

[1] For the sake of greater clarity we may perhaps be permitted to return for a moment to the (here as elsewhere) more transparent sexual life of the man.

mutatis mutandis, to an even greater extent as regards women. Although the more noisy and striking manifestations of jealousy usually come from men (in virtue of their greater tendency to violent and criminal action) nevertheless observation seems to show that jealousy in its minor manifestations acts perhaps more continuously with women, producing "cattiness" and other small acts of hostility, which often tend effectively to stifle the more delicate forms of social feelings almost before they are born. Assuming, as we have done, that women are really in certain respects more monogamously inclined than men, this is what we should expect, so that this tendency to monogamy renders them under both heads—positive and negative—less homosocial than men.

(4) This last factor of a psychological nature is, however, often (especially under present-day conditions) powerfully reinforced by other factors of a sociological nature. Among these is the circumstance that women have, or (what amounts to the same thing for our present purpose) are supposed to have, more to gain by marriage than have men. The congratulations which we shower upon the bride are, other things equal, more wholehearted and sincere than those which, for reasons of courtesy rather than conviction, we bestow upon the bridegroom. We sometimes talk of a man getting "caught" or "trapped" into a marriage, a phrase we seldom think of applying to a woman. Legal actions for "breach of promise" are as a rule only brought by women against men, not by men against women. All these facts imply that we regard marriage as a greater benefit to the woman than to the man. The implications of this attitude are seldom made explicit. It seems, however, to be vaguely felt

that, whereas in marriage a woman has attained the most essential conditions of her well-being (a husband, whose duty it is to provide her with a home and children, together with the increased prestige and dignity that the married state confers), the man on his part, while perhaps acquiring the advantages of a more comfortable domesticity, is sacrificing the advantages of the greater freedom—sexual, social and professional—which the bachelor enjoys. Such an attitude —in some ways perhaps all the more powerful because unacknowledged—necessarily tends towards increasing the desire of women for marriage and therefore adding to the anti-social influences connected therewith, particularly the factor of jealousy and competition among women, a factor the importance of which is perhaps increased by a knowledge of the circumstance that women outnumber men in many of the more populated parts of the earth.

(5) This brings us to a further sociological factor which perhaps outweighs all others both in obviousness and in real importance, i.e. that woman's work, both in civilized and primitive societies, is often of a relatively unsocial nature as compared with man's, in the sense that it brings her into contact with fewer and less varied companions. Even in quite uncultured peoples, the important masculine activities of war and hunting involve social co-operation to a much greater extent than the more feminine activities of agriculture, the preparation of food and the care of children; and throughout the ages women's activities have tended— naturally, as it seems to us, and in accordance with a certain biological inevitability—to retain a relatively domestic and unsocial character. Work within the home undoubtedly provides in many cases far fewer

opportunities for the arousal of social feelings, and the formation of social sentiments towards wider groups of fellow-beings than do the more varied and gregarious activities of men. For this reason, if for no other, women would probably have failed to develop the social and gregarious traditions to the extent that men have done.

(6) The anti-social tendencies resulting from women's economic connection with the more purely domestic forms of work are often reinforced by the still further restriction of women's interests and activities resulting from male jealousy. If for economic reasons "women's place is in the home," men have often endeavoured to make this domestic tie even closer and more rigid than it need be, in order to keep their women from contact with other men. The further restriction of women's outlook through this cause has of course reached its extreme development in certain Oriental cultures, but there are few times and places where it has not played a certain part, and beyond all reasonable doubt it constitutes a potent factor in diminishing women's capacity for social behaviour—a factor the influence of which tends to add itself to the effects of those we have already considered.

VII

THE INCREASING SOCIALITY OF WOMEN

While it seems impossible to dispute the real significance of (at any rate) the last few factors dealt with in the preceding section, it will probably have already occurred to the reader that under present-day conditions the influence of some of these factors is tending to diminish. This seems to be especially and most directly the case as regards our fifth factor (the domestic preoccupations of women). It is a commonplace of sociology that the industrial revolution has to a considerable extent done away with many of the domestic tasks in which women were previously engaged and has at the same time opened up many previously non-existing avenues of activity outside the home. As a result of these changes women's work has tended to approximate to men's, in so far as opportunity for social interests is concerned. This change in the nature of women's work has extended from the industrial to the professional spheres, and there are to-day relatively few walks of life which remain in the exclusive possession of the male sex. In the course of the change, too, women have become "sex conscious"—*i.e.* aware of their peculiar needs and interests, as distinct from, or opposed to, those of men, and the various branches of the "feminist" movement have often afforded striking manifestations of women's new-found capacity for homosocial co-operation that has resulted from this change.

The principal change affecting the nature of women's work has brought with it various important subsidiary changes which affect certain of the other factors that we have considered. Thus there is obviously taking place a corresponding diminution in the strength of our fourth factor (the greater importance of marriage to women). The fact that women have now open to them a great number of commercial and professional activities—suited to all degress of culture and ability— renders them (economically, psychologically and sociologically) less dependent upon marriage than was previously the case; so that this important difference between the attitude of the two sexes towards marriage is tending to diminish. It is beginning to be realized that marriage may involve a sacrifice for women similar to that which it involves for men. Indeed, in so far as women take their professional work seriously (and do not regard it merely as an economic or psychological stop-gap until such time as the more important and satisfying career of marriage can begin), it is clear that the sacrifice required of women may be much greater than that required of men; inasmuch as both sociological tradition and biological fact make it more difficult for them to continue "outside" interests after marriage than it is for men. It even looks as though the conflict between the, to some extent irreconcilable, claims of the professional and marital careers in the case of women were likely to constitute one of the biggest sociological problems of the near future.

The greater freedom of women due to their extra-domestic activities has also brought about a diminution —perhaps we might almost say an abolition—of the artificial barriers to social life in the shape of compulsory seclusion and restraint imposed by masculine jealousy (our sixth factor). Here, as elsewhere in the course of social development, external restrictions have to some extent been replaced by internal moral control; the husband of to-day places reliance in the faithfulness of his consort and in the respect of other men for the marriage tie rather than in an endeavour to prevent his wife having any but the most superficial relations with others of his own sex. The prevalence of this attitude has indeed brought it about that (in contrast to the general antagonism between monogamy and sociality, which we discussed under the heading of factor 3 in the last section) marriage may, in the case of a woman, remove, rather than impose, obstacles to social intercourse. The mechanism at work here is in general similar to that which we already considered in dealing with homosociality and homosexuality; in both cases the inhibitions against the more extreme manifestations of sexuality are felt to be so efficient that inhibitions affecting the more superficial relationships involved in social intercourse can be appreciably relaxed, with a resulting marked increase in social freedom. Thus it comes about that many a woman finds— somewhat to her astonishment—that not the least of the benefits of marriage consists in an easier and less impeded social relationship with men in general. Being excluded as a sexual object for men other than her husband, she can more readily be looked upon as a fellow-member of society, the twin anti-social effects of sexual desire and of sexual inhibition no longer making themselves felt to the same extent as formerly.

VIII

THE PREDOMINANTLY HETEROSOCIAL DIRECTION OF WOMEN'S SOCIALITY

It is interesting to note that these influences making for a more developed social life on the part of women appear on the whole to be manifesting themselves in an increase of heterosociality, rather than in an increase of homosociality. There has for instance been no great enthusiasm for women's clubs, which are still far less numerous and flourishing than men's clubs. Women's clubs too are in general less exclusively homosocial than are men's clubs. Most women's clubs admit men visitors quite freely, rather as though the members soon grew tired of being confined to one another's company and were glad to welcome the presence of the opposite sex. A less ready hospitality is accorded to women in men's clubs, where they still seem to be regarded somewhat as intruders, where they are often confined to one or two rooms specially set apart for this purpose, and where the members introducing them are looked upon to some extent as indulging in behaviour calculated to detract from, rather than to add to, the social amenities of the club. In general the big homosocial organizations of women seem to have been formed only under the stimulus of a strong sex antagonism, such as that which came into existence during the campaign for women's suffrage in the years preceding the Great War. In the absence of such a stimulus the social life of women seems to prosper more in the company than in the absence of men. The homosocial life of men, on the other hand, seems to be much less dependent upon the factor of sex antagonism (though this is, as already indicated, *to some extent* implied in most male homosocial organiza- tions), and there would appear therefore to be still some influences tending to make the homosocial life of men more psychologically gratifying and more sociologically important than that of women. The fact that the recent changes making for the greater sociality of women are on the whole more sociological than psychological in nature suggests that these in- fluences still working in favour of a greater homo- sociality in men are chiefly psychological and are per- haps to be identified with the earlier of the factors mentioned in Section VI, *i.e.* the lesser Narcissism of men, the lesser permeation of male homosociality with sexual (not "aim-inhibited") elements and the less marked tendency of men towards monogamy, with the lesser liability to jealousy that this entails (our previously mentioned factors 1, 2 and 3 respectively).

But although men seem to enjoy a greater homosociality than women, there can also be no doubt that the increased social life of women, tending as this does in a heterosocial rather than in a homosocial direction, is slowly but surely making in some degree for a replacement of homosociality by heterosociality in men. Men's clubs are no longer what they were, and among the chief reasons for their decline is the preference of the younger members for other institutions, public or private, where both sexes contribute to the social life. It is true that such institutions are still struggling with a difficulty from which the homosocial club is free; the difficulty, that is, of steering a middle course between the Scylla of excessive permeation of the social life with gratifications of a sexual kind and the Charybdis of uncomfortable social restraint due to the fear or inhibition of sexual desire. Our modern dance clubs and our more expensive restaurants, regarded from the social point of view, seem to suffer from the former evil; the more staid forms of "cock and hen" club and the social gatherings of our great co-educational institutions suffer rather from the latter. A student moving (as the present writer did some twenty-five years ago) from one of the older universities of England, whose members were—at that time—all of the male sex, to one of the newer co-educational universities, could scarcely fail to become aware of certain subtle elements of embarrassment and restraint which made the social life of the newer institutions less effortless and satisfying than that of the old—an element which upon analysis appeared to be due largely[1] to a certain uneasiness affecting the relations of the two sexes. But there are indications that on the whole this difficulty due to restraint is gradually being shaken off. A comparison of the social life at this newer university at the present day with that of the same university a quarter of a century ago reveals a quite appreciable increase of heterosociality — a lesser segregation of the sexes and a freer social intercourse between them; thus exemplifying, as it seems, the general present tendency for homosociality (particularly male homosociality as the more important form) to be supplanted by heterosociality, the change being due for the most part to the increased social activities of women, which have taken a predominantly heterosocial form.

IX

THE RÔLE OF THE FAMILY IN THE FORMATION OF SOCIAL RELATIONSHIPS

In defining (in Section I) the meaning of the word "social" for our present purposes we purposely excluded any reference to that small but biologically, psychologically, sociologically and economically, most important group of human beings constituted by the family. It is now time however to consider very briefly the relations between the family and the larger "social" groups, in so far as these relations are of importance for our present purpose.

[1] There are obviously other important factors which complicate the situation, such as the collegiate and residential systems, the more influential historical traditions, the greater social (" class ") homogeneity, and above all the easier topographical circumstances enjoyed by the older universities.

Of the four main characteristics of social relationships, as distinguished from sexual relationships, that we enumerated in Section III, viz., greater "aim inhibition" (to use Freud's term), persistence, identification and diffusion, the second and third (persistence and identification) are found in the family relationships to an even greater extent than in the social relationships, and affect to a large extent all members of the family group in their attitude to one another. The first characteristic—"aim inhibition"—on the other hand differs most markedly according to the particular family relationships involved; for many purposes it may be said to be absent as between husband and wife, but affects with quite exceptional degree all other family relationships, in virtue of the incest inhibitions, which play such an obviously important part in many anthropological and sociological phenomena, and which psycho-analysis has shown to be no less important psychologically. Thus with the single but important exception of "aim inhibition" between husband and wife, the first three of our distinguishing "social" characteristics are possessed by the family in a very high degree; to this extent the family might appear to be an institution which works strongly in favour of "sociality" (and against "sexuality"). Very different however is the case with regard to our last characteristic —that of diffusion. It is clear that family relationships in themselves make for a concentration of interest and affection—not indeed upon a single individual—but upon a circle that is very small and intimate as compared with the wider and more diversified surrounding "social" groups—such groups as friends, schoolmates, workmates, fellow-clubmen, fellow-townsmen or fellow-countrymen. It is because of this lack of the element of diffusion that the family has so often been looked upon with suspicion and disfavour by reformers (from Plato onwards) who have had in mind the welfare of larger social groups, who have wished to see the individual identify his interests with these larger groups, and who have seen in the narrower and more concentrated family ties one of the most serious obstacles to this goal. Of recent years, however, certain writers, of whom McDougall is perhaps the most eminent, have expressed the view that in normal development the antagonism between the family and the wider social groups is not necessarily permanent, but represents rather a certain (perhaps inevitable) stage of development. They have pointed out that interest in, love for, and identification with, large groups (especially groups such as can only be conceptually apprehended, such as "the nation" and, still more, "mankind") imply a relatively high level of psychological achievement, a stage which can only be reached through intermediate stages in which interest is directed to smaller and more easily apprehended groups, among which smaller groups the family appears to be the most primitive, most natural and most fundamental. This view is, it may be noted, in harmony with the psycho-analytic doctrine of displacement and sublimation, according to which the development of interest proceeds by a series of relatively small steps from the more "natural" and instinctive to the more complex and cultured; and psycho-analysis itself has indeed provided much evidence to show that interests do in fact proceed from the family to wider social groups in the way that is suggested.[1]   There is therefore much to be said in

---

[1] The present writer has endeavoured to collect and review this evidence in detail in his *Psycho-analytic Study of the Family*.

favour of the view that the family sentiments constitute a useful — perhaps indeed an essential —
stepping-stone on the way to the formation of the
social sentiments.

On the other hand, psycho-analysis has shown, and
perhaps with even greater clearness, that there does
exist in certain ways a real antagonism between family
sentiments and social sentiments, and that, when the
above-mentioned process of development fails to take
place and the family sentiments remain in sole possession
at an age when they should normally have given place
to sentiments connected with larger social groups, there
may result a very serious lack of social interest and
feeling, a lack which may appreciably decrease the
social value of the individual.

It thus appears that both those who have seen in
the family a menace to the development of social
feeling, and those who have seen in it an important,
perhaps essential, condition for this development, have
to some extent right upon their side. The psychological data at present available justify us in assuming
that, as the earliest and most natural of all groups of
individuals, the family plays a very significant part in
the first arousal of the desires and feelings that bind
an individual to his fellows; feelings that, after a series
of "displacements", may later on become operative in
the formation of wider "social" bonds. But it is also
clear that, in so far as these feelings remain permanently
attached to the narrow circle of the family, they may
prevent the formation of the more diffused sentiments of love for our fellow-men that are of the
essence of the higher kinds of social interest and
behaviour.

F

X

THE VARYING NATURE OF THE PSYCHOLOGICAL RELATIONSHIP BETWEEN THE FAMILY AND SOCIETY

In these remarks we have considered the family only in its relation to modern life. A somewhat wider view may be obtained by contemplating the relations between the family and society in historical perspective. Unfortunately the materials for a detailed history of the family are not to hand and many aspects of the matter are subjects of considerable controversy. Nevertheless a few main phases of development possess a certain degree of clearness as regards their chief outlines, and a brief consideration of these phases would appear to be of interest for our present purpose.

There seems to be no doubt that the family is biologically the most primitive of groups. As to how and at what time the larger social groups developed from this primitive group there is much difference of opinion. According to Carveth Read,[1] the larger group arose through the adoption of a flesh diet and the habits of hunting in order to acquire it—a change that took place at the pre-human level and that indeed (according to him) accounts for the development of the essential human characteristics, both bodily and mental. On this view the foundations of the family and of society respectively are to a large extent distinct and independent; both biologically and psychologically, the relations between members of the family and between members of the herd have but little to do with one another. This would agree well with (though it does not necessarily imply) the view that

[1] *The Origin of Man.*

the sexual, the parental, and the gregarious tendencies correspond to separate and independent instinctive mechanisms.

According to some other views the larger social groups arose more directly from the family group in a manner that was largely determined by feelings and desires aroused within the family circle itself. Most notable of these views is the Darwin-Atkinson-Freud hypothesis, according to which the social sentiments grew chiefly among the younger males on the dual basis of hostility to the father of the family and of sexual abstinence (owing to the father keeping the females for himself); the psychological ties that are operative being in the nature of an identification on the basis of a common misfortune and of a common desire to be revenged on the father and to usurp his privileges (particularly his sexual privileges).

It will be observed that on both of these views the social feelings and the social ties originated among men as distinct from women, so that they both suggest that the greater sociality of men is a fact of great antiquity, one that is not peculiar in any way to historical times or civilized conditions.

Whatever view of the origin of society we may adopt, there seems to be a pretty general agreement that at the earliest stages the wider social groups were relatively unstable, fleeting and unorganized, as compared with the more permanent, archaic and stable unit of the family—monogamous or polygamous— governed by a single powerful male. From this stage onwards we may, largely following the guidance of Wundt,[1] distinguish three main further phases of development of the family and of society.

[1] *Elements of Folk Psychology.*

In the first of these, which, adopting Wundt's convenient terminology, we may call the Totemic Age, there is a higher grade of culture and a much more elaborate social organization than in the stage of the primitive family. Indeed, the family, in so far as it depends on blood relationships, recedes very much in importance in favour of the more definitely social unit of the clan; while the different clans in their turn are often knit together in wider units. This is the period of totemism and exogamy, of the classificatory system of relationships, of strong matriarchal tendencies and of avuncular rather than paternal jurisdiction. In many ways this age presents an amazing contrast to that which went before, and indeed it is true that the connection between the two has never been satisfactorily described and remains at best extremely hypothetical. In the view of Freud and of those other psycho-analytic writers (notably Róheim) who have followed him in his excursion into anthropology, the social arrangements of this age may be said to represent a triumph of reaction against the primitive jealousies of the Oedipus complex that were so prominent in the earlier period. Group marriage and exogamy provide means of sexual gratification without arousing the fiercer anti-social elements of competition that the sexual passions are otherwise apt to bring about. At the same time, as Reik[1] has so convincingly shown, secret societies and initiation ceremonies are inspired by an attempt at reconciliation between successive generations, between the father and the sons. Important vestiges of the previous condition of greater antagonism between the elder and the younger men are to be found, however, in the institution of the Men's House, to which we

[1] *Op. cit.*

have already referred. In so far as the younger men live together (though now no longer always in sexual abstinence), while the older married men live with their families, there is a perpetuation of the earlier state of affairs, the social life being still fostered (as Schurtz[1] has pointed out) by the younger rather than the older men. On the whole, however, it seems as though at this stage mankind were succeeding (at the cost, it is true, of much serious restriction of their activities in the shape of taboos) in reconciling their sexual with their social needs, and that in so doing the family as based on blood relationships were giving place to wider social structures.

These earlier social organizations were, however, not destined to develop smoothly and continuously into larger and more civilized societies, probably because they were not capable of being adapted to the more numerous and complexly related groups of individuals that improvements in material culture gradually rendered possible. Instead of the supersession of the family by the clan that is characteristic of the Totemic Age, we find in the next stage that the family has once more become important; though co-existing now with a much wider organization constituting the state or nation. This is the age of the patriarchal family,[2] under the influence of which we are to some extent still living. The revival of the family has brought with it a recrudescence of many of the difficulties and anti-social factors that are perhaps inevitably connected with family life; difficulties of which we do not always willingly become aware and the full magnitude of which has only been revealed by psycho-analysis[3];

---

[1] *Op. cit.* [2] Wundt, *op. cit.* 311 ff.
[3] Cf. the previously cited work of the present writer.

difficulties the general nature of which we have, so far as they concern us here, already dealt with in the previous section.

But though the family is at present more important than it was in the Totemic Age, we seem now to be actually in a stage of transition to another period—corresponding in many ways to Wundt's period of "development to humanity"—in which the influence of the family is once more declining and giving place to that of wider groups. Industrialism, compulsory schooling, increased facilities for travel, the cinema, broadcasting—influences such as these bring the individual into contact with social life outside the family in a way that was not possible 100 or even 50 years ago, and correspondingly free him from the exclusive prestige and authority of the family circle. This increase of social influence seems to be manifesting itself as regards groups of all kinds and sizes. On the one hand there are springing into existence innumerable clubs and societies for purposes of social intercourse or for the furtherance of the most varied aims—social, literary, sporting, political, scientific; while on the other hand a sense of community of interests between members of different classes, races and nations is developing the more conceptual aspects of social life. The loosening of the bonds of family and the diminution of *patria potestas* are of course especially notable in the case of women, who, as was before noted, are now entering into social life in a way that was formerly confined to men. In fact, as has been strongly argued by Müller Lyer,[1] there seems to be a pretty close correspondence between the social position of women and the general development of sociality, as

[1] *Phasen der Liebe*, pp. 180 ff.

distinct from the hegemony of the family; a correspondence which may seem at first astonishing in view of what we have found concerning the important part in social development played by associations between men, but which can nevertheless be seen to be in harmony with economic facts and which is less startling also when considered in relation to a further correspondence to which we must now turn.

This further correspondence consists in a tendency for an increase of sociality (and a concomitant decrease in the influence of the family) to be accompanied by a certain increase in the freedom of sexual relations. The Totemic Age, as we have seen, although imposing immensely strong taboos in some directions, provided relatively easy means of sexual gratification in others— much easier means than existed at an earlier period, if we accept the Darwin-Atkinson-Freud hypothesis, which is the most explicit on this point; this age did indeed seem to provide temporarily a successful solution of the conflicting claims of jealousy and sexuality. In the present age of transition something of the same sort seems once more to be happening. In recent years, concomitantly with the decline in the power of the family and the increase of social life, there has gone on a change towards a freer and more tolerant attitude towards sexual life and sexual problems. We have already seen that a marked feature of recent developments in social life is an increase of heterosociality. But this increase of heterosociality (as a part of the general increase of sociality as a whole) has also been accompanied by an increasing freedom in certain aspects of heterosexuality. How is this fact (and the corresponding changes involved in the earlier transition to the Totemic Age) to be reconciled with the apparent general antagonism between sexuality and sociality from which we set out? It seems that there must be here at work some important factor which we have so far failed to take adequately into account, and which may necessitate a substantial revision of the terms in which this antagonism should be stated. It looks as though, in concentrating on the opposing aspects of sexuality and sociality, we had failed to do justice to certain features which they have in common.

A very brief consideration, however, of some of the facts that we have already passed in review seems to show that the nature of the common features can to some extent be inferred from much that we have already said, especially in so far as these common elements are of a negative order. It would seem that many of the factors antagonistic both to sexual and to social life depend largely upon jealousy and the sense of exclusive possession. Jealousy and the sense of possession are quite obviously among the most fundamental causes of sexual inhibition and restraint. According to Freud's and Róheim's hypothesis of the *Urhorde*, it was the jealousy of the head of the primitive family ("the jealous sire")[1] which imposed sexual abstinence upon the younger members of the horde. In modern times and in the patriarchal family it is clear that it is the authority of the head of the family which ultimately provides the sanctions operative in producing many of the sexual inhibitions. But if jealousy is one of the prime causes of restrictions on the sexual life, it is also a force that is highly destructive

---

[1] The influence of the family authorities is made very clear in Freud's doctrine of the Super-Ego, according to which this authority is incorporated as a permanent moral sanction within the mental structure of the individual.

of social life, through the mutual suspicions and dissensions to which it gives rise. According to Freud,[1] indeed, the restraint and control of jealousy is one of the important conditions of social life. The whole social system of the Totemic Age may be said to aim to some extent at the elimination of jealousy; it is an age characterized by a relatively feeble sense of individual possession. In modern times the increase of social life has also been accompanied by a less jealous surveillance over the younger members of the family, particularly the girls; while socialism, which aims at the abolition as far as possible of all forms of individual possession, has, as we have already incidentally reminded the reader, been usually associated also with a tendency to the denial of possessive rights over family or sexual partner. Jealousy and exclusive possession and authority are, however, facts of great importance in giving influence to the family; it is the *patria potestas*—the power of the head of the family over the junior members —which ultimately knits the family together into a powerful and important group. In the variations of jealousy and sense of possession we may see, therefore, the chief reason why the development of family authority is inimical to sexual or social freedom and why these latter (sexual and social freedom) tend to vary inversely as the former (jealousy, sense of possession and influence of the family).[2]

[1] *Group Psychology*, p. 86.
[2] See also the article " Some Problems of Jealousy " in the present volume.

XI

THE CO-OPERATION OF SEXUAL AND
SOCIAL INSTINCTS

In the light of these considerations with regard to certain factors which make for a positive (instead of a negative) correspondence between sexual freedom and sociality, we may now return to our main theme, the antagonism of sex and society, dealing by way of conclusion with the more fully fledged sentiment of sexual love, the condition of "being in love" as distinguished from more ephemeral and sensual desires.

The manner in which "love" (in this sense) acts anti-socially is plain enough; it is through the intense concentration of interest and affection upon a single individual. A passion which will enable us to "count the world well lost" so long as it is satisfied might seem at first to make us utterly unconcerned about the thoughts and feelings, weal or woe, of our fellow-beings other than the one we love. We have already done full justice to the antagonism between "love" and sociality that undoubtedly exists in virtue of this concentration. There remain to be considered, however, certain, perhaps less conspicuous but none the less important, ways in which "love" aids rather than impedes the development of social sentiments.

In the first place romantic "love" involves a certain degree of inhibition of the sensual elements of sex attraction—a character which, as we have several times observed, it has in common with the affections that are involved in social ties. How far the social sentiments may actually benefit from this "aim inhibition" involved in romantic love it is difficult to say. For the most part it would appear that the "aim inhibition" is used for the purposes of the "love" itself. Nevertheless this "aim inhibition" does not apply merely to the relations with the loved object, but to some extent affects the whole of conduct, and it is therefore quite possible that it may facilitate the formation of social sentiments, in so far as preoccupation with the loved object leaves over the necessary time and energy for the formation of such sentiments. In any case, however, it is important to remember that the social sentiments and the condition of "being in love" both imply the capacity for "aim inhibition"; both may profit by this capacity and both may tend to strengthen it.

In the second place "love" undoubtedly involves a certain limitation of egoism and of Narcissism. As Freud has pointed out,[1] the idealization of the object implies a drawing off of the Narcissistic libido attached to the Super-Ego, in extreme cases the object actually taking the place of the Super-Ego.[2] This withdrawal of Narcissistic libido leaves the Ego "unassuming and modest" and less egoistic than it would otherwise be. The Super-Ego as projected on to the loved object is often more powerful than in its unprojected form. The desire to please the loved object, to become worthy of it, may lead to a great increase in susceptibility to ethical influences, *i.e.* the conduct of an individual, though perhaps still less gregarious than before being in love, is now more definitely in accordance with social standards. He may in fact become a socially more valuable person than he was before.

Closely connected with this is the fact that, in a

---

[1] *Group Psychology*, pp. 74 ff.

[2] A doctrine which has certain interesting features in common with that of Danville (*Psychologie de l'Amour*).

good many cases, "falling in love" appears to endow the whole of life with a higher degree of value and seems consequently to liberate fresh sources of energy, which directly or indirectly may be used for social ends; in such instances there may result, in fact, a great improvement in the capacity for sublimation. The conscious reasons for this increase of energy may be somewhat various, ranging from the economically conditioned desire to make marriage possible to the abstract and idealistic wish of the lover to make himself more worthy of his (idealized) love object through the practice of virtue. In some cases, however, there seems to result from "falling in love," not only an increase of socially valuable, but an increase of socially directed interest and affection. Though loving in a concentrated manner (or more correctly, just because he is loving in a concentrated manner) the lover has also at his disposal more "diffused" love for social purposes.[1] Thus, in certain lovers, the love they feel for their idealized love object seems to irradiate some

---

[1] Although in other cases the results of "falling in love" may of course be of negative social value, as when a lover loses interest in his social occupations and his work and "wastes" his time in melancholy pining for his mistress, or else, when under the influence of an unscrupulous love object, he allows himself to be instigated to directly anti-social acts. It would seem that in the first case there is something akin to the impoverishment of the Ego that takes place in grief and melancholia, while in the latter case the love object has actually taken over the functions of the Super-Ego (cp. Freud, *Group Psychology*, p. 75). In the cases of positive social value considered in the text, it would seem as though both the Super-Ego and the Ego of the lover had been strengthened and harmonized through the projection of the former on to the loved object, with a consequent enrichment of the whole personality. Perhaps the process of harmonization is brought about by the fact that the instinctual desires are now actually directed towards the very person upon whom the Super-Ego has been projected ; so that the attitude of the Id to the Super-Ego is much more wholly one of love than is usually the case (for although a certain amount of love is perhaps always present in this attitude, the element of hate is usually also prominent).

of its effulgence, so that even the rest of mankind appear as more lovable than they were before. In such cases the joy of being in love makes the lover feel at peace with all the world; he feels he can adopt no other attitude than that of love towards a world that is made glorious by the presence of his loved one. Every kind thought and generous deed in relation to humanity at large is at once inspired by, and directed to, the central object of affection—a condition of affairs which has obviously much in common with certain religious states in which the love of God stimulates, and overflows into, the love of humanity.

Astonishing, and even paradoxical, as these cases may at first appear, they probably represent only specially striking instances of what is at bottom a general tendency of great importance; a tendency which seems to point to a certain deep-lying connection between the sexual and the social feelings. The overflow from sexuality to sociality can indeed, it would appear, sometimes be detected by direct introspection, and this apart from any special condition of "being in love." Thus at least one man of good introspective ability and experience has informed me that he was able to detect a sexual element underlying both the pleasure of actual social contact with his fellows and the interest and enthusiasm which he felt for social reform. As he put it: "It is the love of (real or imaginary) women which seems to contribute a good deal to the joy I may experience from social gatherings and a good deal of the energy which I throw into speculations, plans, or actions, aiming at social progress. In the guiding concept of a better and happier humanity I find something that produces a sort of vague and diffused sexual excitement. Humanity for me could appropriately enough be symbolized in the form of a beautiful woman."[1]

Quite apart, however, from such direct introspective evidence there are at least three sets of facts which indicate the existence of some such general tendency:

(1) The change in, and increase of, sexual feeling at adolescence coincides with an emergence of a deeper social feeling, greater capacity for altruistic sentiments and a greater interest in ethical and social problems. As one writer has well put it: " With the dawn of adolescence comes the recognition of a larger life, a life to be lived in common with others, and with this recognition the desire to sustain the social code made for the common welfare."[2]   Since the monumental work of Stanley Hall, the existence of such a connection between the final development of the sexual tendencies at puberty and the fuller appreciation of the nature of social relationships has indeed become something of a commonplace.

(2) If normal sexual development brings with it an increase in the strength and delicacy of social feeling, it would seem very probable that the converse is also true, for a certain blunting of the finer social feelings has been frequently supposed to accompany any gross interference with proper sexual development.   Thus eunuchs have often been credited with a lack of the

---

[1] It seems quite probable that similar motives entered into the work of certain social philosophers, *e.g.* Comte and J. S. Mill. Cf. too the words " She stepped into the centre of that dream of world reconstruction that filled my mind and took possession of it all " which H. G. Wells puts into the mouth of one of his heroes, at a moment when this hero—and all his fellow-men—are filled with a great uprush of social feeling. (*In the Days of the Comet*, Book III, ch. I—a story that is largely concerned with our present problem.)

[2] E. M. Darrah, quoted by Stanley Hall, *Adolescence*, II, p. 394.

higher social virtues of courage, faith and loyalty, and with an unenviable capacity for low cunning and intrigue.

(3) But apart from any such physiologically or anatomically conditioned failures of development, psychopathology has of recent years shown very conclusively that sexual maldevelopments of a purely functional nature are also frequently connected with social deficiencies. Neurosis, due to conflicts over sexual tendencies and connected with sexual repressions, usually brings social disabilities in its train; the victim of such a neurosis being as a rule both less agreeable and less valuable socially than the normal person; whereas when (through psychotherapeutic measures, through a favourable change in outer circumstances, or through a combination of both these influences) the sexual life has become satisfactorily adjusted, the patient's social behaviour usually exhibits a corresponding improvement.

All these facts showing concomitant variations of sexual and social feelings would seem to be more easily reconciled with the psycho-analytic view that sexual and social interests spring ultimately from the same source than with the view that we have to do with separate and independent sources of instinctive energy. At any rate they show clearly that there are certain common factors which affect advantageously or disadvantageously both sexual and social adjustments, and which therefore tend to create a positive rather than a negative relation between the two kinds of behaviour. Furthermore, if we accept the almost universally held view that sexual interests are, both ontogenetically and phylogenetically, the more primitive and fundamental, we may conclude that a satisfactory development of the social sentiments is to a large extent dependent upon the healthy development and function of the sexual tendencies.

We are now in a position to see the whole problem much more clearly. From our present point of view it seems as though the antagonism between the sexual and the social interests, from which we started out, is one that, in spite of its great importance, is relatively superficial, in the sense that it can only come into being at a certain fairly advanced stage of development. Even if we refuse to accept Freud's libido theory of the social relationships (which, in spite of the difficulties of detail that it raises, does from our present standpoint undoubtedly seem best to fit the facts), we must at least agree that both sexual and social sentiments have certain fundamental factors in common and that, in particular, social sentiments will flourish most, not where there is a deep-seated inhibition of the sexual functions, but where there is a diversion of interest from the sexual to the social field after the sexual functions are already well developed.[1]

Furthermore, we have already seen in the earlier sections of this paper that much of the apparent conflict between the sexual and the social interests is not so much connected with the sexual tendencies as such, but rather with the socially disruptive jealousies to which these tendencies give rise. This does not make the antagonism in question any less intense, but it does give us a better comprehension of its real nature and at the same time indicates in what way it can be

[1] In this respect the antagonism here in question is very similar to that more fundamental antagonism between self and sex, which was considered in a paper by the present writer " On the Biological Basis of Sexual Repression and its Sociological Significance," *British Journal of Medical Psychology*, 1921, I, p. 225.

diminished; namely, by reducing the part played in sexual life by the desire for exclusive possession. And it would seem indeed that the trend of present development lies in this direction. Corresponding to the lesser claims of the family to possess and control its individual members—a matter with which we have already dealt—there is on the whole a tendency towards a reduction of jealous watchfulness on the part of lovers also. In marriage the element of affection is coming to be considered of greater importance than the element of possession and exclusive privilege. We can at least appreciate in theory that the altruistic element in love—that element which seeks the well-being of the loved object—is of greater value than the egoistic element through which pride is satisfied by possession of this object. We can even sympathize with the extreme case in which a lover might forgo his claims upon the person whom he loved, because he considered that the welfare of this person would be better served by abandoning his claims—a position which would seem contemptible and ridiculous when judged by a standard of ethics in which possession rather than love played the leading rôle.

This overcoming of the insistence upon exclusive rights in love is one of the most difficult tasks [1] with which the development of sexual ethics is confronted. It is quite possible that the task may not be successfully

---

[1] The task here is parallel to that of reducing the claims to exclusive possession in the sphere of economics. (Cf. what was said above about the connection between social reforms on the one hand and marriage and the family upon the other hand.) In both cases men have to realize that, by abandoning exclusive claims, they gain more by the furtherance of social feeling and co-operation than they lose by the rigid insistence upon rights, the benefits of which are often problematical so long as they are seriously challenged by others.

G

accomplished—at any rate for many generations yet to come. But if it is accomplished, it seems clear that the antagonism between the claims of sex and of society will be very much reduced.

XII

SUMMARY

(1) There exists a certain antagonism between the manifestations of sexuality and those of sociality.

(2) There are two chief views as to the nature of the principal instinctual energies involved in the sexual and social tendencies respectively. According to one view the instincts of sex and of the "herd" are separate and distinct. According to the other (Freud's libido theory) the instinctual energies involved are at bottom the same, the social tendencies being only special differentiations of the sex instinct.

(3) Following Freud we may distinguish four important ways in which social tendencies differ from sexual tendencies:

(i) The absence of the sensual element ("aim inhibition" according to Freud's theory);

(ii) Greater permanence;

(iii) Greater identification;

(iv) Greater diffusion, *i.e.* reference to a larger number of individuals.

Of these the last appears to be the most constant and important.

(4) All four of these factors serve to make social relations between members of the same sex ("homo-

social" relations) easier than social relations between members of the opposite sex ("heterosocial" relations).

(5) Male "homosociality" is nearly always more developed than female "homosociality." Among the reasons for this may be:

(i) The anti-social influence of the greater Narcissism of women;

(ii) The fact that with women homosocial relations are more tinged by, and more easily pass over into, homosexual relations than with men;

(iii) The fact that women are more monogamously inclined, this tending to produce both less dispersion of affection and greater liability to jealousy;

(iv) The fact that women have more to gain by marriage than men, this also tending to increase jealousy;

(v) The fact that women's work gives less facilities for social relationships than does men's;

(vi) The seclusion of women (due ultimately to male jealousy), which has often powerfully reinforced the influence of the two previous factors.

(6) Under present-day conditions the social differences between the sexes are tending to diminish, and women are coming to take a larger share in social life.

(7) The increased social life of women is, however, on the whole taking a heterosocial rather than a homosocial form, and in so doing is tending to increase the heterosociality of men also.

(8) The institution of the family is in some important ways antagonistic to that diffusion of interest which social sentiments demand. The family sentiments may, however, act as useful—perhaps essential—stepping-stones to social sentiments, though when too persistent

they may prevent the adequate formation of social sentiments.

(9) In the course of successive ages there appear certain changes in the influence of the family as compared with that of the wider social environment. The family is probably the most primitive and natural social unit, but in what, with Wundt, we may call the "Totemic Age," the family based on blood relationship receded very much in importance as compared with the clan; in some ways a satisfactory compromise seems to have been arrived at between jealousy and sociality. Later, the family once more became important, though at the present day it is again giving way to an increasing social influence. Sociality implies a limitation of jealousy and of the right of exclusive possession over children or sexual partner, whereas the family is to a large extent founded on the *patria potestas*. Since sexual inhibitions also ultimately depend indirectly upon jealousy, there is here at work an influence which tends to produce a *positive* correspondence between sexual freedom and the preponderating influence of larger social groups (and a negative correspondence between sexual freedom and preponderating influence of the family). [This influence is therefore opposed to the antagonism between sexual and social tendencies, from which we set out.]

(10) Moreover, romantic sexual love aids rather than impedes the formation of social sentiments in that:

(i) It demands some degree of "aim inhibition";

(ii) It demands a limitation of egoism and Narcissism;

(iii) It may lead to increased sublimation;

(iv) It may lead to an overflow of love on to others.

This last fact points to a certain deep-lying connection between sexual and social feelings—a connection that is also indicated by the simultaneous reinforcement of both at adolescence and by the fact that organic or functional disturbance of the sexual life also disturbs the social life.

In the light of these considerations it would seem that the antagonism between sexual and social feelings only concerns the direction of energy at a relatively high level and that the satisfactory development of the social sentiments to some extent presupposes and depends on the healthy function of the sexual tendencies.

As we have seen, too, much of the antagonism is really connected, not with the sexual trends as such, but with jealousy, and the extent of the antagonism is perhaps being diminished at the present time by a decline in the importance of the element of possession in the sexual life.

SOME PROBLEMS OF JEALOUSY [1]

IT is generally admitted that jealousy is a factor of great importance in social and sexual life, though opinions as to its ethical and social value differ widely. To some it seems the principal breeding-ground of hate and suspicion, an element that is largely destructive of the finer bonds of social feeling, while to others it appears to be one of the chief forces that produce cohesion and stability in the family, and therefore ultimately also in the larger organism of society. The former view is held predominantly by those who hold "progressive" or "advanced" ideas. We are not here primarily concerned with this thorny question of the ethical evaluation of jealousy, but rather with a psychological analysis and description of its causes and its inner nature. And yet it is scarcely possible to keep ethical considerations altogether in the background; they continually obtrude themselves, both because of the inevitable prejudices on the part of the investigator and as corollaries that are ever and again suggested by our psychological conclusions. It may be well therefore to confess at the outset that the present writer belongs to the school which sees in jealousy an evil rather than a good.

A superficial examination of jealousy in its psychological aspects seems to show that it can be split up into a number of paired opposites; in the first place there are, on the one hand, the feelings of frustration

---

[1] A paper read to the British Sexological Society.

caused by the loss—real or feared—of a loved object; and, on the other hand, the feelings of inferiority caused by wounded self-esteem. In the second place, there is grief caused by the loss; while at the same time there is hostility towards the person who has caused it. In the third place, this hostility may be directed to the loved object herself (it will incidentally be convenient to employ one form of personal pronoun throughout and to consider the jealous person as the male, but this is due merely to the deficiencies of language), or to the person who has alienated her affections.

It does not require any very deep analysis to show that in any of these aspects of jealousy there are apt to be purely psychological reactions which are greatly in excess of those which a true and purely reasonable estimation of the loss would justify. Thus, so far as our first pair of opposites is concerned, it is clear that, looking at the matter from the point of view of real requirements, no one needs the continual presence or affection of any other single person, even in the extreme case of this person being the object of a concentrated and exclusive passion. From the purely objective point of view there should be no resentment if the loved person bestows part of her time, energy and affection in other directions, so long as this does not interfere with the real needs of the lover himself. Even the most ardent lover requires the occasional stimulus of other beings, if only to afford a foil or contrast; and many persons are so constituted that periods of solitude are not unwelcome. With regard to the wounding of self-esteem, it is very clear that this cause of distress is artificially fostered by ideas concerning property or "honour," and in this case it is easy to prove that such ideas are largely dependent on current sociological conceptions. Where ideas of honour or economic interest are not fostered by the artificial structure of society or the prevalent system of social ethics, these aspects of jealousy practically disappear; as is shown in those numerous societies where men will willingly, and without any feeling of resentment, lend their wives to others, whenever social customs so dictate (and will take offence if such offers are rejected).

Recent psychological researches, and more especially those of the psycho-analytic school, have thrown considerable light on the deeper motives of these "unreal" elements of jealousy,[1] and it would seem that proper appreciation of these motives is essential to an adequate understanding of the part played by jealousy in social life, and an adequate treatment of the many moral problems connected therewith.

From the very start, psycho-analytic doctrine has emphasized the great importance of jealousy in early life. Jealousy is an essential component of the famous Œdipus complex, which results from the inevitable tendency of the young boy to look upon his father as a rival for the affections of his mother; and, as is now well known, psycho-analytic workers have tended to look upon subsequent situations involving rivalry as in some sense merely repetitions of the original "triangular situation"—repetitions which derived their emotional significance from the fact that they stirred up passions which were originally aroused in the young child by his relation to his parents, and which led to the development of a mental attitude which has never been completely outgrown or overcome. Freud regards

---

[1] See especially Ernest Jones, "La Jalousie," *Revuè Française de Psychanalyse*, 1929, III, p. 228.

the Œdipus situation as giving rise, not only to the "nuclear" components of the neuroses, but also to some of the most fundamental conflicts underlying social life. In so far as his brilliant espousal of the Darwin-Atkinson hypothesis of the origin of human society is justified, it is not surprising to find that jealousy has constituted everywhere one of the essential problems in the organization of social and sexual life. If it is true—as psycho-analysts believe—that the Œdipus complex of infancy is seldom, if ever, altogether outgrown, and that it is, in powerful if unsuspected ways, a determinant of conduct in later life, then our understanding of the great importance of the "unreal" elements of jealousy in adults is carried one stage farther; while if it is true also that the revolt of the sons against the primal father was an event of supreme importance in the development of human society— —as the Darwin-Atkinson hypothesis maintains—then we can also understand that the reactions to jealousy constitute important differentiating elements in the various forms of human social organization. We see at once why jealousy is valued highly by those who uphold the patriarchal form of organization, and is regarded as an evil by those who look upon society as a band of revolutionary brothers rather than as an enlarged family under the dominion of a "jealous sire."

However this may be, light is thrown on jealousy in the second place by the consideration of certain features of the child-mind itself (as distinct from elements which are dependent on the early social situation of the child). The very young child is less tolerant of loss, frustration and renunciation than is the adult, partly because the inhibiting mechanisms which make renunciation possible have not been developed, and partly because the child has not yet learnt that renunciation may be merely temporary. The adult is consoled by the idea, which experience has taught him, that temporary frustration is a rule of life, but that gratification will eventually recur. To the child, lack of immediate gratification implies all the tragic consequences of a permanent deprivation. It is as though the inability to secure his mother's breast at any given moment carried with it the implication that his mother was permanently lost to him, and he himself therefore destined to die of hunger. This inability to distinguish between temporary and permanent loss seems to be, to some extent, a general characteristic of the unconscious and the primitive levels of the mind. Thus, in spite of conscious awareness to the contrary, the neurotic may feel after orgasm that his potency is lost for ever; and the savage in the autumn believes that the sun will never again shine high in the heavens as in summer, unless certain magical rites are undertaken to ensure this otherwise unlikely event. The persistence of this attitude in the individual's unconscious mind may give rise to a neurotic fear of loss, and a desire for exclusive and permanent possession. As a recent author has put it,[1] the attitude of the child for his mother is very similar to that of the monogamist to his wife. Like the mother, the wife must always be present and available, for otherwise she will, to his unconscious mind, be permanently lost.

Such a love implies of course that the needs of the lover can be satisfied by one woman only, and this

---

[1] R. Money-Kyrle, *Aspasia*—a book which is written from a point of view very similar to that adopted in the present paper and to which the present author is considerably indebted.

leads us to a third important factor—the existence of specialized or concentrated love, or quite simply "love," if we use the term in its popular sense. It has been truly, though somewhat cynically, said that being in love consists in greatly exaggerating the difference between one woman and all others. In virtue of this monopolization of all charms by a single individual it is of course impossible for others to replace her; her loss is really irreparable, while the unique evaluation of her lasts, and the existence of other persons of her sex is an entirely irrelevant matter. It is clear then that the psychology of specialized love is an important factor in the origin and maintenance of jealousy; in its absence there would logically be no cause for jealousy, so long as other possible love objects were available. For obvious reasons we cannot here enter into the great and complicated question of the psychology of "love," a question on which psycho-analysis, more perhaps than any other method, has also cast some light. We may, however, point out one element that seems to be especially important for our present subject, namely the endeavour to find in the loved object the unrealizable ideals of infancy. Freud, Rank and others have convincingly shown the very strong tendency that there exists to idolize the *imago* of the parent, the tendency to perpetuate the notion of perfection which, in a sense, the parent really possessed in the eyes of the young child. One of the most difficult processes of education consists in realizing the imperfections and limitations of one's parents, a realization which in many cases is only rendered possible by the creation of an imaginary substitute for the real person whose claim to perfection can no longer be upheld. This craving for a perfect being may show itself in many ways. It may lead to the creation of gods and goddesses; or (and this is what concerns us here), it may lead to the notion that there somewhere exists the perfect man or woman, a completely satisfactory love object, the infantile idea of the parent carried over into adult life. To some extent this notion of the perfect being is applied to every person who is sincerely loved; hence the loss of this person is indeed a tragedy, a repetition of the loss experienced in childhood. But it is easier to imagine the qualities of perfection in a being who is unknown or unpossessed than in one with whom we are actually intimate. Hence the love object whom we might possess, but do not, is more apt to be endowed with these qualities than the one we actually possess; and if we have possessed her and she is taken by another, her desirable qualities thereupon all too easily become accentuated. Thus to many of us, the wife or mistress of another man seems better than our own, while the one whom we have actually possessed seems more desirable after we have lost her. In this way then the illusion of an unrealizable ideal greatly fans the flames of jealousy.

While, on the one hand, the widespread presence of this ideal increases the difficulty of loss, to many it may also actually increase the likelihood of such loss. In virtue of the fact, already mentioned, that a relatively unknown person can more easily appear to incorporate the ideal than a known one, the attractions of other men's women are apt to undergo a spurious enhancement. The search for the ideal, constantly disappointed and constantly renewed, is one of the major factors leading to a restless promiscuity, so that its presence in many members of the population may give rise to a multitude of Don Juans, each depriving the others of their would-be spouse, each, in so far as he is a successful robber, being disappointed, but, in so far as he is robbed, being inconsolable for his loss.

We have here a number of important factors rooted in infancy, which, if not outgrown, make for jealousy in later life. That these factors are not more often outgrown is, to some extent at any rate, due to the circumstance that our original attitude to children and young persons often prevents the development of alternative reactions and substitute gratifications for the infantile desires and fears in question. Normal development implies the acquisition of a number of new and, as we are wont to say, "higher" reactions, in the place of the simpler, cruder and more instinctual tendencies of the child—this acquisition of new tendencies being described by psycho-analysts as the process of "displacement." But the earlier displacements are themselves often crude and unpolished, and therefore liable to meet with adult disapproval rather than encouragement; and if, as a result of this disapproval, the alternative outlets are excluded, there is "fixation" at the original stages and objects of desire, even though this fact may be to a larger extent unrecognized owing to repression.

The very earliest tendencies of the child are predominantly oral in nature, corresponding to the fact that the mouth is the principal zone of interest at this state of development. The child endeavours to find a substitute gratification for the absent nipple by sucking his thumb, a practice which is usually frowned upon by nurses and mothers; and many other oral habits of the child meet with similar discouragement, often with reason (for the child tends to put all objects indiscriminately into his mouth), but not always so. At a slightly later stage, the anal interests of the child meet with even greater signs of disapproval, for the adult is utterly incapable of understanding the child's natural attitude towards his excrements. When the genital regions of the body and the genital activities in turn become the predominant centre of interest, here too the child meets with frustration and reproof. Owing to the notion that children are, or should be, pure and innocent, infantile masturbation is met with threats and scoldings, sometimes even by physical violence or constraint; and anything in the nature of erotic play or curiosity between children usually meets with the severest punishment and disapproval.

The atmosphere of the school is in this respect similar to that of the nursery, and as far as possible proscribes all sexual activities and interests up to, and during, adolescence. Indeed, it has been said with justice[1] that the moral intolerance of educators is directly proportional to the normality of the impulse that is condemned. Fetishisms and definitely neurotic substitutes for sex are merely laughed at or ridiculed. Nocturnal pollutions are regarded as perhaps inevitable evils. Masturbation is pursued with threats and admonitions, but is not as a rule made the subject of a too severe inquiry. Homosexual passions may be tolerated so long as their sensual aspects are not too blatantly paraded, though, if it becomes impossible to ignore them, they are sternly dealt with. But the harshest methods of all are reserved for the manifestations of heterosexual love, which are the natural accompaniments of adolescence.

Even in the freer atmosphere of post-school life, our present social régime places innumerable difficulties in the way of sexual manifestation, but does all it can

[1] Money-Kyrle, *op. cit.*

to emphasize the compensation which may ultimately
be secured in the one legitimate and socially recognized
sexual outlet of monogamous marriage. Since marriage
is thus regarded as the only recompense for a long
series of privations and frustrations, it is not surprising
that the privileges and rights connected with this
institution should be jealously preserved with an
intensity of passion which does not always correspond
to the satisfactions actually secured. We can perhaps
realize the situation more easily if we compare it with
an imaginary analogous situation in another sphere.
An author to whom we have already referred [1] suggests
what is in some ways an illuminating comparison
between sex and food. "Jealousy" he says, "may be
a natural impulse, but so is greed. Yet greed is largely
outgrown while jealousy increases. Imagine a people
kept for a great portion of their lives in a state of semi-
starvation and at length only permitted to eat their fill
on condition that each chose some one dish they were
not previously allowed to taste, but which should henceforth be reserved for them as their sole sustenance for
ever. The prevailing vice of such a people would
certainly be greed, for they would be excessively
envious of each other's food and exceedingly jealous of
their own. Those who were not engaged in stealing
scraps from someone else's cupboard, would be occupied
in savagely defending their own hoard, even if they do
not want it."

Our present attitude towards sex therefore encourages
jealousy:—in the first place by consistently placing
difficulties in the way of natural development and
thus producing a fixation upon the early stages; and
in the second place by stressing the compensatory

[1] Money-Kyrle, *op. cit.*

importance of an institution in which exclusive possession is by tradition and precept an all-important
element. The individual is thus encouraged to retain
that intolerance for the temporary loss of a loved object
which is characteristic of infantile life. The toleration
which is not shown to the infant, when it demands
that its mother shall be in constant attendance and
shall not divide her attention between himself and
his father, brothers and sisters, is, as it were, eventually
and belatedly shown to the married adult, who, it is
supposed, can legitimately demand of his spouse that
she shall have no other lover than himself. And yet
on *a priori* grounds it might perhaps have been thought
that the child, who has not yet learnt to bear temporary
frustration, might be deserving of greater tolerance
than the adult, who has had ample opportunity of
finding out that no one person is necessary to him all
the time. The infantile attitude has in fact been carried
over to the adult institution. There may be, under
certain circumstances, adequate justification for the
insistence on exclusive possession, but here we are only
concerned with the matter as it appears from the directly
psychological point of view.

All the facts which we have hitherto considered deal
with a general attitude which is recognized in consciousness, although the ultimate roots of this attitude
have only recently been explained. Psycho-analysis
has shown, however, that there are still other factors,
which are for the most part scarcely recognized in
consciousness at all. Two of these factors must be
mentioned here. In the first place, jealousy is greatly
strengthened by the unconscious envy of the greater
freedom which the existence of an aberrant impulse,
real or imagined, in a spouse implies. All married

people are continually tempted to unfaithfulness. If, for instance, the husband suspects the wife of giving way to this temptation, in thought or deed, he unconsciously envies her the greater freedom that she has won for herself through this emancipation. The corresponding impulses in himself are thereby strengthened, and a satisfactory way of dealing with the situation is to condemn, and demand punishment for, the offender. This is a mechanism which is not confined to marital morality, but plays an important part in our whole attitude towards crime or other infringements of social law and custom. As psychoanalysts have shown,[1] one of the reasons why we so insistently demand punishment for offenders is that they have stirred up temptations to corresponding behaviour in ourselves. It is as though we were tempted to ask ourselves why these offenders should have gratified themselves in an unsocial way, while we have not; why should not we also allow ourselves the same indulgence? Social justice is felt to be infringed if the law and custom breakers have obtained forbidden enjoyments which we have denied ourselves. Justice must be carried out by infliction of pain to compensate for the illicit gratification and (what is perhaps even more important) in order that we may reassure ourselves that such illicit gratification is not really safe. Our repressions, which were threatened by the action of the criminal, are thus reinforced, and we can continue to inhibit our own delinquent impulses. In the same way, it is only through the insistence on the penalties—legal or moral —incidental to unfaithfulness that the monogamous spouse can himself continue in the narrow path.

[1] See, for instance, Alexander and Staub, *The Criminal, the Judge and the Public.*

H

The other factor described by psycho-analysis is of an even more surprising nature, but the evidences for it are overwhelming. From one point of view however, it can be regarded as merely a startling instance of the unconscious envy to which we have just now referred. It has been regularly found that excessive jealousy of the paranoiac kind is always associated with the repression of homosexuality.[1] Unfaithfulness in a wife means that she has relations with another man. The husband, in virtue of his homosexual tendencies, identifies himself with his wife, and thus vicariously exposes himself to homosexual indulgences. Homosexual desires are, however, in such cases repressed, and not as a rule permitted to invade consciousness, even in this vicarious form. The moral condemnation of his own desires for a male love object (a condemnation which is responsible for the repression) is extended to these desires as they exist, or are imagined to exist in his partner. In his unconscious mind he envies her her opportunities, and would like to find himself in her place; but, since this attitude is subject to repression, the fiercer his unconscious temptations, the more suspicious and intolerant will he become. Psycho-analytic research is showing more and more that this factor of unconscious homosexuality, while predominant in pathological cases, also plays a rôle of no inconsiderable importance in many cases of what we regard as normal jealousy. The presence of the homosexual element can indeed be shown very clearly in certain instances where a husband's wild and savage jealousy, leading to a desire to kill his wife or her lover, will alternate with the idea that her relation with another man is an

---

[1] See, for instance, Freud, " Certain Neurotic Mechanism in Jealousy Paranoia and Homosexuality," *Collected Papers*, Vol. II, p. 232.

intensely fascinating thing, which he will get her to narrate in every detail afterwards, or which (better still) he will himself observe from some secluded corner.

Owing to the presence of this homosexual element, jealousy may often exist, as it were, in two dimensions; either offending party may play either rôle. At the more conscious level, the man is grieved because the woman of his choice has given her favours to another. At a deeper level he may be equally perturbed, because this other man has manifested love to the woman rather than to himself. This is especially liable to be the case when there already exist bonds of friendship and affection between the two men concerned.

It is not surprising that an affect of such depth and complexity should be capable of causing intense suffering to all concerned; primarily to the jealous person himself, and indirectly to the object of his passions, whose love he fears to lose. In this sphere it is more than ordinarily difficult to distinguish the abnormal from the normal. The acute forms of jealousy seem almost inevitably to acquire something of a delusional nature, so that the victim sees confirmation of his suspicions in the most harmless acts or words; both his own life and that of his wife or mistress are rendered miserable by needless complaints, innuendos or restrictions.

In certain cases too the jealous person's sufferings may be increased by the sadism or hostility of others. The simplest hint may suffice to arouse his ever-ready suspicions, and he is thus exposed to any torment which those about him, exasperated by the unnecessary complications that he causes, or hostile to him for any other cause, may choose to inflict.

Summarizing the general nature of jealousy, as it emerges from the foregoing considerations, we may say perhaps that it possesses four principal characteristics:—

(i) Jealousy is to some extent fantastic and "unreal," in that it is based upon supposed needs which do not correspond to genuine requirements. It is based on unnecessary fears; it rests upon the false assumption that the presence and ministrations of the loved person are continually needed—an assumption which seems to be founded on the infant's attitude towards its mother. It thus contains a large quasi-neurotic element, and is to this extent a sign of weakness rather than of strength. The person who had learnt to recognize his real needs and their limitations, and who had sufficient confidence in his own ability to ensure their satisfaction when required, would suffer comparatively little from the pangs of jealousy. At any rate, he would only suffer from them in so far as his real needs rather than his imaginary and potential needs were in danger of frustration. And this would mean a very significant diminution of the power of jealousy.

(ii) Jealousy arises in circumstances which are to some extent a repetition of the original situation which gave birth to the Œdipus complex, and itself indicates often enough a fixation at this stage of mental development. Those who have largely outgrown the Œdipus complex are less exposed to the ravages of this emotion.

(iii) Some forms of jealousy may depend upon unconscious envy of the—real or supposed—greater freedom of the person whose conduct has aroused the jealousy.

(iv) Jealousy is often related to the existence of homosexual tendencies in a repressed state, and in its extremer forms seems almost invariably to be so related.

(v) On the sociological side jealousy is associated with the morality proper to a patriarchal system in which the rights of the father extend to the presence and affections of certain other individuals who are in a very real sense his property. In such a society the infringement of the father's or husband's rights in this direction are liable to arouse a lively sense of outrage or inferiority, which can only be appeased by vengeance. Moreover, our social and educational traditions tend greatly to enhance the jealousy springing from this source.

Jealousy is, therefore, a true and natural sanction of the patriarchal system, and is looked upon as reasonable and laudable by those to whom this system seems the keystone of social life and civilization. It is, on the other hand, largely incompatible with a system of liberty, equality and fraternity, in which every individual has some right to the free bestowal of his or her affection and in which this right is regarded as of greater importance than the right of property. Jealousy is naturally and inevitably disruptive of this latter system, which cannot be so tolerant of exclusive privileges over individuals or over property. Quite rightly, therefore, the upholders of this system condemn jealousy, as an emotion which is harmful to society and which inflicts unnecessary suffering and frustration.

The present age is one in which social and economic circumstances are inevitably emphasizing the desirability of wider social bonds and correspondingly diminishing the importance of the family and the range of *patria potestas*. It is, therefore, an age in which the problems of jealousy are of very real importance. Indeed, in its wider bearings, jealousy is connected with some of the most important of contemporary social problems. Modern psychology has shown that the feelings which were originally directed to the family or to the sexual life may be displaced on to the larger groups or institutions of society. There is much evidence to show that the envy that one social class will show towards another may be, psychologically speaking, derived from envy that was originally of a sexual nature, *i.e.* the jealousy which a social class living in relative poverty harbours towards the wealthier classes may be, to a large extent, derived from the feelings with which the son regards the privileges of the father. The original object of desire, the possession of a loved person over whom the father had exclusive rights, may find a substitute in a new object of desire, such as wealth or rank or power, which, as in the case of the originally desired object, appears to be unjustly monopolized. Here too we find again the characteristic feature of jealousy, which we have already stressed, *i.e.* that it is based, not so much upon real need,[1] as upon the objection to sharing of privileges with another. In so far as this displacement of sexual jealousy to the social and economic field is a *vera causa*, we must suppose that sexual frustration and its associated jealousy plays a much larger part in the political sphere than has been hitherto suspected.

The complexes that find their expression in jealousy may also play a part in international politics. The individual citizen regards his country in the same way as he regards his wife (and ultimately his mother, as the word "motherland" testifies). Both have to be protected from the unwelcome attacks or attentions

---

[1] Of course I do not for a moment wish to suggest that there may not be reasonable grounds for envy based on purely economic factors. I only mean that these factors are in many cases not psychologically adequate or ultimate.

of outsiders, outsiders who in the last resort symbolize the father. The citizen's honour too is equally involved in both cases. In the latter instance, however, the situation is sometimes more complicated, in that, especially in monarchistic or autocratically governed countries, the country may be looked upon as the privileged possession of the king or ruler. Here, as in some other instances in the political sphere, the individual sides with the father and protects the father's privileges against the hostile manifestations coming from his own unconscious desires. In this case, the citizen's own unconscious tendencies are symbolized by the enemy.

Those who are of the opinion that, in both its social and individual manifestations, jealousy is predominantly harmful at the present time will naturally seek to discover what are the most hopeful ways of diminishing the arousal and development of jealousy. If our previous considerations are justified, we may suggest that there are six main ways in which we may hope to diminish the incidence and strength of this emotion:—

(i) We must endeavour to prevent fixation at the infantile stage of thought, at which the child demands the permanent presence and affection of its mother. Unfortunately we are still too much in the dark concerning this obscure and remote period of mental development to offer as yet any very hopeful suggestions in this sphere. It is a sphere, however, on which child psychology may ultimately throw some light. From what we know, it seems likely that oral frustration, as the psycho-analyst would call it, has much to do with the development of a neurotic sense of insecurity.[1]

[1] See, for instance, Edward Glover, "Notes on Oral Character Formation," *International Journal of Psycho-Analysis*, 1925, VI, p. 131.

If this is so, we may reasonably expect that adequate and regular nutrition would be the most likely means of abolishing the fear of permanent deprivation. It may even be that a certain pampering of the very young child may be beneficial, though probably the problem will turn out to be a good deal more complicated than this simple suggestion may lead us to suppose.

(ii) It is clear also that we must endeavour to prevent as far as possible the formation of an unduly strong Œdipus complex. The jealousy of the child should not be needlessly and gratuitously aroused. This is one of the few precepts on which psycho-analysts have all along insisted, and it seems not altogether unlikely that in future we shall learn to be much more tolerant of jealousy in the child, and less tolerant of it in the adult than we are at present.

(iii) We must also endeavour to prevent fixation at the Œdipus stage, and this, as we have seen, may mean the removal of many of the restrictions and threats which at present encumber the sexual development of the child. A greater freedom to indulge in the sexual activities proper to each stage of development is almost certainly the best, and perhaps the only, means of avoiding those elements of jealousy which spring from an unconscious identification of later situations with those of early life within the family.

(iv) Freer sexual development implies also the adoption of a more liberal attitude towards homosexual tendencies, and conversely it would seem that the absence of jealousy and the implied ability to share the affections of the loved object with others of one's own sex depends upon the ability to love these latter persons; though this love need only be of a sublimated, or, as Freud would say, an "aim-inhibited" kind. It is the kind of love which permits of identification, so that in sharing the affection with others we are still enjoying it, though in a vicarious form. When the homosexual tendencies are too sternly repressed, this identification becomes impossible, and we are deprived of this vicarious compensation for our own loss.

(v) At the more conscious plane, we should endeavour to discourage the notion of property in love and seek to dissociate self-respect from the existence of exclusive rights. This task can perhaps be made easier if we bear two facts in mind. In the first place, that it is impossible to ensure exclusive affection, but at most to prohibit the manifestations of affection to others; so that the demands of jealousy are necessarily to some extent based on a delusion and a sham. In the second place, that the ideas of property and honour associated with jealousy are sociologically connected with the patriarchal tradition; a tradition that, in its turn, is somewhat out of harmony with modern social and economic trends, which are inevitably diminishing the importance and solidity of the family as the fundamental social unit.

(vi) Last, but not least, we must stress the radical importance of a healthy sexual life for adults. We should lay more emphasis on the positive benefits and satisfactions of love than on the dangers and wickedness of infringing taboos and exclusive privileges. It is clear that the bearing upon sexual morality of many new factors in the sexual and social life of our times has been inadequately thought out. Birth control, the question of the legalization of abortion, and the control of venereal disease, are three such factors, the ethical implications of which are difficult to overestimate. But these are clearly important themes deserving of extensive treatment on their own account. Superstitions and taboos apart, modern science is diminishing many of the more "rational" causes of sexual inhibition, while the modern ethical outlook, in stressing the right to the fullest individual development independent of sex or social station (to some extent even independent of age), removes many other moral justifications for jealousy that formerly existed.

Jealousy is undoubtedly a tendency of the human mind which is inevitably aroused in some degree by the very conditions of our existence. Nevertheless, with the help of a reasonable education and an enlightened social order, it can be so checked and modified as to be rendered comparatively innocuous—if we so desire.

MAURICE BEDEL'S *"JEROME"*—
A STUDY OF CONTRASTING TYPES[1]

I. *Bedel's Statement of the Problem.*
II. *The Contrasting Types Examined.*
III. *The Underlying Principle and its Applications.*

I

BEDEL'S STATEMENT OF THE PROBLEM

A FEW years ago Maurice Bedel published a novel,[2] which was awarded the Prix Goncourt and aroused considerable amusement and some indignation in at least two countries. It was translated into English and soon attained the respectability of the conventional but almost incredible publication figures that decorate the title pages of all French best sellers. The amusement and indignation, as also perhaps some other features of the novel's career, were due to the fact that, under a slight veneer of literary irony, it expounded, in trenchant but truthful fashion, two conflicting points of view— points of view so wide in outlook that they may fairly be called philosophies. These philosophies are more- over of no mere academic interest, but have on the contrary the liveliest practical importance, inasmuch as they distinguish the main underlying trends of the

[1] Reprinted from *The Psycho-analytic Quarterly*, 1932, Vol. I.
[2] *Jerôme, 60° Latitude nord* (Nouvelle Revue Française). English trans- ation : *Jerome, or the Latitude of Love* (Duckworth), from which the quota- tions in this paper have been taken.

present day erotic life (and therefore also to a large extent the social life) of the already mentioned countries. As the philosophies in question have seldom if ever been explicitly treated in modern psychological literature, we may perhaps be permitted to take Maurice Bedel's book as a text for a preliminary orientation of the problems concerned—problems which, as we shall see, reveal themselves even to casual examination as of wide import and considerable complexity.

Jerome, the hero of the novel, who also gives it its title, a young and successful French playwright, is on his way to Christiania (as the city was then called) to superintend the production of one of his own plays. He is of an ardent and romantic disposition, given to innumerable short-lived love affairs, each of which promises the happiness it does not give, but for a moment fans to a fresh brilliance the fitful flame of his idealistic passion.   In fact, he is a typical, and, we must admit, a very charming, specimen of the Don Juan type, in which love can be satisfied only by a perpetual succession of new objects.   Such satisfaction had not been lacking, for in his short career he had been as successful in love as in literature, and, so far as the former was concerned, "it had as yet brought him no other disenchantment than a certain monotony of success." The novel which bears his name is devoted to the history of the affair which occupies him during his trip to Scandinavia—an affair which, we are given to understand, makes a more profound impression than most others.   The object of the affair, a young Norwegian girl, Uni Hansen, presents in many respects the greatest possible contrast to Jerome, a contrast which, as the background of the novel makes us realize, is in a sense intended to epitomize the cultural aims and

viewpoints of the respective countries of the two protagonists. Uni represents the extreme of childish
common sense, matter-of-factness and naïveté. As
seen through her eyes, life seems to be a relatively
straightforward, obvious business, with few com-
plexities to worry over and little room for sentiment
or romance. In her relations with Jerome, as in
her dealings with other men, the sexual elements
seem at first to be subordinated (to Jerome himself
exasperatingly subordinated) to those of common
humanity; but, when sex appears, it is as "natural"
and straightforward as the rest—a matter about which
it is unnecessary to fuss or bother, remote as it is alike
from ecstasy, romantic longing, or disgust. There is
not an atom either of coquettishness or prudishness in
Uni. To Jerome on the other hand a certain sexual
obsessiveness is the very spice of life; quite clearly
and consciously, it constitutes the driving force of all
his thoughts and doings. He is continually seeking
situations which will provide him with the necessary
romantic setting for a declaration of love; situations
in which Uni behaves as though she were a child
ignorant of all the subtle meanings—nay, even of the
very purpose—of the intricate sexual game which so
largely occupies Jerome's thoughts and feelings. But
when at last he does make clear his meaning, she
responds with a directness that is as disconcerting as
was her previous camaraderie; a directness that brings
into startling relief another correlated feature of Jerome's
sexual life, namely—his need for secrecy, intrigue and
complication, in all matters of the heart and of the
senses. To Uni a declaration of love means an engagement, and an engagement means an obvious, open and
unashamed indulgence in sexual relations, which, if

sufficiently agreeable to both parties, will in turn mean
marriage—a marriage which itself shall last while
mutual inclination persists, but shall be dissolved
without recrimination or protest by either party, should
the one or the other tire of the relationship or be
attracted elsewhere. To Jerome such simplicity is
not merely incomprehensible, it is devastating; for,
while on the one hand it betrays a childish lack of
reticence and of discretion that is definitely repellent,
on the other hand it seems to rob love (and with it life)
of all that is most fascinating and attractive, all that is
most worthy of the wits and emotions of a cultured man.

In due course the inevitable happens. While in the
unfamiliar snows of Norway, the romance endures,
through the very piquancy of its incomprehensibility
and strangeness; but soon the pair are dispatched by
the relatives of Uni on a sort of unofficial honeymoon
to Copenhagen. Even on the journey the conflicting
points of view continue to assert themselves, as when
Jerome engages two sleeping compartments—to him
an obvious proceeding in the interests alike of decency
and of adventure, but to Uni's simpler mind merely a
useless extravagance and inconvenience. Arrived in
their hotel at Copenhagen Uni retires to the bath-room
only to ask Jerome to bring her the eau de Cologne.
Jerome is seized with an anxiety attack, says he cannot
find the missing bottle, and afterwards, when Uni
comes into the room and proceeds to put into practice
an elaborate system of massage and gymnastics (in the
literal sense), he becomes absorbed in the changing of
the guard, which is providentially taking place in the
square below him. During the day, in the, to him,
more familiar atmosphere of a larger and more cosmo-
politan town, his infatuation for Uni declines rapidly,

in correspondence with a reawakening of the desire for
ever-new adventures—for which indeed the Danish
capital appeared to afford every facility. In the evening,
in a bedroom scene in which Jerome further demon-
strates his incapacity to carry out what seem to Uni the
obvious duties of a fiancé, Uni, puzzled, but retaining
her imperturbable good humour, suggests that Jerome
does not know these duties, and offers to teach him
them, saying that she is already well instructed from a
previous honeymoon of this description (incidentally
with the man who taught her the system of massage
and gymnastics, which had proved such a trial to
Jerome in the morning). Jerome, appalled both by the
revelation and the prospect, locks the communicating
door between the two rooms. In the morning Uni
utters neither reproach nor disappointment, but, in
the intervals of renewed gymnastics, is full of sympathy,
good advice and practical solutions of their difficulties.
"*Comment vous allez, pauvre petit?*" were her first
words as she offered him a frank handshake. "You
ought to do a lot of gymnastics," she advises him,
"You're not a strong man." "I!" said Jerome, irritated,
"I assure you that in France . . . !" Uni stopped in
the middle of her exercises and, looking at him with a
sort of pity, she pronounced simply and decisively the
fatal words: "Jerome, you talk a lot, but you never can
do anything. And when the time comes for you to do
something, you can only weep. You're not the kind of
fiancé for me. I give you back your freedom." Jerome
had hoped for tears, entreaties and pathetic scenes
rather than for advice on matters of physical culture.
Nevertheless, this frankness and matter-of-factness
awakes in him a certain common element of human
sympathy, from which, however, all sexual factors seem

to be excluded—and thus they part good friends, he to return to Christiania to explain matters to her mother and to wind up his affairs in that city before definitely leaving Scandinavia; she to stay with friends in Copenhagen for a short visit before (as the reader is left to imagine) entering upon a new engagement with her former fiancé, who had once again proposed himself in that capacity on the eve of Jerome's and Uni's departure for Denmark. To complete the picture, it may be added that, as a last generous gesture, Uni had offered to plead his cause with a girl friend of hers at Copenhagen, whom they had met the previous day and for whom Jerome had expressed admiration—a gesture which, we are told, made Jerome all the more regretful to take leave of a comrade who pushed self-sacrifice so far as to offer him her best friend in exchange for herself.

Having thus indicated, very briefly and with omission of all detail, the main theme and characters of the story which we have taken as our text, we may be permitted to make a few further quotations from this text, with a view to making still clearer and more vivid the problems of which it seems to be a statement.

Jerome recognizes from the start that Uni is at once more childish and more masterful than the other girls with whom he had philandered. But then he expected something in the nature of a new experience on this journey to a new country, a country which his imagination had already lavishly endowed with romance. Perhaps too, the absence of some of the more usual distinctively feminine traits and of the sexual responses to which he was accustomed, constituted a challenge to his character as a successful sexual hunter and at the same time awoke certain masochistic features of his nature.

At the termination of one of their first meetings, we are told, "she grasped his fingers with a vigour in which he recognized more comradeship than was pleasing to him. It was a boy's handshake. But as he left her, he reflected that a descendant of the. Vikings could not have the manners of a village maiden, that Queen Zenobia, Atalanta and Nausicaa had been both tender and fearless; and moreover, since Norway was a land of forests, it was fitting that her daughters should wear the likeness of Diana." With regard to his masochism, which delighted in the self-tormenting aspects of his loves, we read: "The blow he received from his first meeting with Uni the evening before on the deck of the *Jupiter* had left its bruise, and in sly complicity with the weakness of his nature, he hoped it would spread until it had taken possession of him."

The general impression of a certain childishness and innocence which the Norwegian women made on Jerome is well conveyed in the following short passage: "Their candid eyes, their doll-like complexions, the unconcern with which they wore hats several years out of style, provided him with a kind of pleasure that he missed in the Paris buses. Quite unintentionally he smiled at them as one smiles at a pretty child. Nor did they appear to be offended. They were simple as fountains and as fresh as bathers, without make-up and without mystery."

On Christmas eve, which is a festival that each family celebrates within its own closed circle, to the exclusion of all strangers, Jerome nevertheless arranges to meet Uni for a few moments outside her house. She puts him into the garage where he can shelter from the cold, and brings him from time to time a few delicacies from the family table. Jerome at last experiences some

I

of the delights of a romantic intrigue, but is horrified
at the absence of all air of secrecy or precaution from
Uni, whose occasional expeditions outside the house
seem indeed to arouse no interest in her relatives. In his
desire to make the most of the situation, he endeavours
to read danger and high romance into a situation that
is at most a little ridiculous and undignified. "He
shrank into a shadow among the shadows, a plank in
the fence, like a criminal about to be exposed by the
thoughtlessness of his accomplice. But deep within
himself, he was tasting a keen delight in this danger,
hoping that he might be discovered by the traditional
duenna, pursued by the jealous lover and attacked by
the watch. Fear is an emptying of the will, the delight
of the weak."

This, however, was almost a unique occasion in a
long series of desperately straightforward situations,
which in the long-run, when they had ceased to appeal
by the mere force of their amazing novelty, could only
end by producing in Jerome a peculiar combination of
boredom, terror and disgust. Jerome's habitual values
begin to reassert themselves in the more complex
environment of Copenhagen. "Under the lights of
the restaurant, the pleasures of life had no value unless
they were the result of intricate minute and studied
ingenuities like the steps of this tango. He regretted
that they were not throwing balls of coloured cotton
from table to table, which so facilitates the birth of
intrigues; and that someone did not ask Uni to dance,
so that he himself might invite the little brunette in
the cyclamen dress at the next table. He realized that
he was growing bored with the simple emotions. Uni
on the contrary was noisily happy over trifles."

But perhaps the most illuminating statements of

the two opposing points of view are to be found in
Jerome's conversations with Madame Krag, the mother
of Uni, of which we quote a sample:

MADAME KRAG: ' Love? Why love is when Axel says to all
the world "I love Gerda Josefsen." And when Gerda says: "I
love Axel Hansen." And they are married. It is a straightforward
thing.'
JEROME: 'And if some day Gerda says to all the world, I no
longer love Axel, I love Sigurd, and if Axel says nothing and sees
his children go to live with Sigurd, is that also a straightforward
thing?' (un acte franc).
KRAG: 'Yes, and it is much better than if Gerda slept in Axel's
bed and dreamed of Sigurd.'
'A straightforward thing . . . a straightforward thing . . .'
thought Jerome. 'But love is not so simple as all that. . . .'
"They were passing through the lobby of the theatre at this
moment, under the bristling eyebrows of a bronze Ibsen.
'A straightforward thing,' said Jerome. 'Yes, to be sure. But
still, sometimes. . . . Well, for example, there was Nora in *The
Doll's House*. Now in France she would have been a very good little
wife and wouldn't have broken things up. She would have deceived
her husband with much discretion and propriety. . . .'
KRAG: 'What horrible ideas you have.' "

As already mentioned, Jerome explains the situation
to Madame Krag on his return from Copenhagen.
When she has received his report, their final conversation is as follows:

KRAG: 'In short you failed in all your duties.'
JEROME: 'What!'
KRAG: 'In the pursuit of love you encounter human nature at
every turn, and you imagine that you can settle everything by
shutting your eyes.'
JEROME: 'Should I open them?'
KRAG: 'Yes, Jerome, when the garments of custom fall and the
veils of habit are drawn back. . . .'
JEROME: 'But, madame, these were the veils of a young girl.'
KRAG: 'And wasn't that young girl your fiancée?'
'A mother who reproaches me for having respected her daughter,'
thought Jerome.
"Madame Krag then expounded certain principles of eugenics

which overturned all of Jerome's ideas of engagements. As her premise, she declared that the basis of marriage was truth and that nothing should be hidden between two beings who had chosen each other freely. She could not find words severe enough to describe the custom, prevalent in old civilizations, of uniting two strangers for life, of leading up to the nuptial bed a man in evening dress and a girl hidden behind a veil, of saying to her 'you are his wife', and to him 'you are her husband' before their tastes, their affinities and their physical suitability had been tried out in an honest test.

'Love,' she repeated, 'is a straightforward thing which flourishes in marriage between those two guarantees of personal happiness, betrothal and divorce.'

"Jerome detested this point of view. Can one take guarantees against a sentiment whose dwelling is the sublime? To risk the adventure of happiness with a woman seemed to him a goal sufficient in itself.

'Madame,' said he, 'I am not accustomed to a love that supplies itself with guarantees.'

'You prefer to have it lead to falsehood and treason.'

'That's an exaggeration.'

'And to murder,' she added.

" She left the room abruptly, and returned a moment later, carrying a file that bulged with newspaper clippings.

'Here, read these,' she said, putting them in Jerome's hands.

" He found a collection of those tales that are one of the attractions of the French press and the favourite literary nourishment of the middle classes:

'Jealous lover gashes Mistress: Attempts Suicide' — 'Frightful Vengeance of a Deserted Woman: Abandoned, she throws herself into the Seine with her Child'—'A Drama of Jealousy'—'A Drama of Pistols'—'A Drama of Vitriol.'

'Well,' said Jerome unconcernedly, 'that is what love is.' Madame Krag gazed at him with horror."

II

THE CONTRASTING TYPES EXAMINED

If we seek to summarize the differences between the two mentalities at the descriptive level, we shall arrive at some such list as the following:—

Jerome	*Uni*
1. Complex	Simple
2. Sophisticated	Naïve
3. Adult	Childish
4. Romantic	Matter-of-fact
5. Sexual interests continually in the foreground	Sexual interests often subordinated to others
6. High degree of genital supremacy.	Somewhat diffused erotism
7. More masochistic	More sadistic
8. Direct sexual manifestations somewhat inhibited	Direct sexual manifestations uninhibited
9. High degree of sex differentiation	Low degree of sex differentiation
10. Desire for secrecy and intrigue	Frankness
11. Little agreement between social theory and individual practice	Considerable agreement between theory and practice
12. Sense of conventional propriety developed	" Advanced " ideas on propriety
13. Much overestimation of sexual object	Little overestimation of sexual object
14. Much jealousy	Little jealousy
15. Neurotic	No signs of neurosis

The first five items on this list would seem to be so obvious as to require no immediate comment. We may merely remark that Jerome's complexity and sophistication strike us as adult characteristics and that Uni's simplicity and directness seem in comparison to smack of the childish and the relatively undeveloped—a difference that is in harmony with several other items on the list.

With regard to number 6 it seems clear that Jerome's sexuality is much more under the hegemony of the genital component instinct than is Uni's, this again being, according to psycho-analytical conceptions, more in accordance with the adult pattern. Uni's relatively diffused sexuality manifests itself particularly in her delight in sports and gymnastics (and perhaps also in her general *joie de vivre*). In this matter the author seems to have pointed to an undoubtedly typical difference between the national mentalities that are represented by the two protagonists. In France there is little general *interest* in sport and gymnastics as compared with Britain, Germany and Scandinavia (though there is pretty clearly no lack of *ability* in these directions). Nor was there until recently the enthusiasm for *Nacktkultur* or *Aktphotographie* of the more "harmless" sort, such as, in Germany (until the advent of the Nazi régime) drained off a good deal of libido at a slightly sublimated pregenital level. The greater hegemony of the genital components with the French tends to make such manifestations of diffused erotism appear to them childish and uninteresting, while their own more constant preoccupation with love and sensuality on the genital plane is in turn apt to appear to Northern visitors as a sort of sexual obsessiveness (since only the unmistakably genital is usually reckoned as sexual, so that many manifestations of the more diffused sexuality of the Northern races is apt to escape recognition as such).

No. 7 (masochism—sadism) relates to an important difference in the direction of one of the component instincts. Uni's sadism shows itself chiefly in her muscular preoccupations, and in particular in a trait to which we have not yet referred, namely, her enthusiasm for boxing. Indeed, an admiration for French achievements in this sport is an important factor in her original interest in Jerome, who hypocritically pretends to share her interest in pugilism—a pretence which he has, later on, reason to regret, when he has to submit to a good pummelling at Uni's hands. Whereas Uni's sadism is chiefly muscular, Jerome's masochism—in harmony with the greater complexity of his nature— is primarily psychic. We have already noted the

author's allusion to his satisfaction in the self-imposed
sufferings of love and the "weakness of his nature"
which longed for such sufferings and desired to be
"taken possession of." In the light of recent psycho-
analytic knowledge, we may suspect too that in this
masochism is to be found the explanation of a great
deal that Uni (and with her, perhaps, the reader, if he
is honest) finds complicated and bewildering in Jerome's
nature. The author's reference to a "sly complicity"
in virtue of which sexual desire tends to become mingled
with masochistic pain almost irresistibly suggests
Alexander's formulations [1] concerning the corruptibility
of the super-ego and its conspiracy with the libido to
permit satisfaction to the latter on condition that pay-
ment be made in terms of suffering—a conspiracy that
seems to underlie so many manifestations of neurosis.
If this interpretation is correct, it would seem that the
masochism of the present case is, like that of many
others (as Freud has pointed out), the meeting place
of the instinctual urges and of the inhibitions emanating
from the super-ego, the two opposing tendencies both
finding satisfaction in the same symptoms. Instinct
and inhibition have thus become closely bound together
—the former can only be satisfied on condition that
the latter is also operative: if inhibitions are removed,
instinctual satisfactions are by that very process, as
it were, eviscerated, so dependent have these satisfactions
become upon the overcoming of an obstacle. We have
here, I believe, the most important key for an understanding of Jerome's mentality and of the differences
between his mind and that of Uni, in whom there
does not exist this complex and subtle relationship
between desire and inhibition, and in whom there

---

[1] F. Alexander, *Psychoanalyse der Gesamtpersönlichkeit.*

is much less (if any) dependence of the former on the latter.

These considerations would seem to throw considerable light upon the various other items of the list. They tell us, for instance, something about the nature of the greater complication and sophistication of Jerome as compared with Uni (Nos. 1 and 2). They remind us also that such complication and sophistication, due to the dependence of desire on inhibition, are more characteristic of the adult than the child, so that characters in whom such dependence is marked are apt to appear to us more "grown up" than those in whom it is absent or minimal (No. 3). With regard to No. 4 (romantic—matter-of-fact) we shall surely suspect (a suspicion for which we could find much corroborative evidence) that romance springs from inhibition of the simpler forms of satisfaction and is both dependent on it and expressive of it. Romance deals essentially with the overcoming of obstacles to satisfaction, as a study of any piece of romantic imagination, from the story of the Golden Fleece to the novels of Rider Haggard, will surely show. In the present case, what are Jerome's phantasies of the "duenna," the "jealous lover," and the "watch" but imaginary dangers and difficulties conjured up to satisfy his insatiable need for obstacles, i.e. in the last resort so many projections of his own inhibitions?

With No. 5, however (degree of predominance of sexual interests), we come to a complication—a complication which is perhaps present in the others also, but in which it less imperiously demands our attention. Part of the apparent difference in this respect between the two mental types in question is probably due to the tendency, already noted, to overlook the more diffused

and pregenital constituents of the libido that play a
relatively important rôle in the type represented by
Uni. But this can scarcely account for the whole
difference. A certain obsessiveness in Jerome's sex
life seems to indicate that it has a neurotic element that
is absent in the case of Uni—a neurotic element that is
connected, once again, with the complex interplay of
inhibition and libido. It would seem, in fact, that the
obsessiveness of Jerome's sexual thoughts and desires
is a consequence of inhibition—inhibition that is of
course only partially successful in its aims. We are
here up against the fundamental fact that incomplete
inhibition intensifies desire, giving it at once a strength,
a permanence and a quality that are scarcely to be found
in the absence of such inhibition. It is this fact that
constitutes the main theme and moral of Maurice Bedel's
book; and the chief purpose of the present essay is to
emphasize the far-reaching psychological, sociological
and ethical consequences of this fact.

Turning to No. 6 on our list, (degree of genital
supremacy), the general knowledge at present available
would seem scarcely sufficient to enable us to say what
is its precise relationship to the facts that we have been
discussing in connection with No. 7—whether, that is,
the degree of genital hegemony of the libido is in any
way due to the strengthening of the libidinal elements
through inhibition. That genital hegemony means to
some extent a successful repression and subordination
of the pregenital elements there can be little doubt.
But this repression does not imply so much a strengthening as a redistribution (and concentration) of libido,
and it is not easy to show that any strengthening of
libido occurs in genital hegemony.

When we turn to No. 8, however (degree of inhibition

of direct sexual manifestations), we see that the inhibitions in Jerome's case are not confined to the pregenital
levels but powerfully affect the more direct expressions
of genital sexuality itself. Jerome's anxiety attacks in
Copenhagen clearly point to a feared or actual impotence, the alleged reason for refusing to see Uni
when divested of her clothes—the fear of spoiling the
romantic nature of the whole adventure—being pretty
clearly in the nature of a rationalization. The real reason
is interestingly brought out by a small detail of the
scene. Jerome pretends to be absorbed in the spectacle
of the changing of the guard and in describing this to
Uni he exclaims: "How very curious! the drum major
is lame . . . He's not very lame, but all the same, for
a drum major!" Anything, the author tells us, was
good enough for rescuing his love from a mortal danger;
but nevertheless, here as elsewhere, the "something"
that was chosen was probably not without a psychological significance; for lameness, as we know, is by
no means a rare symbol for impotence or for castration.
His love in fact was in mortal danger from a source
other than that of which the ordinary reader (or perhaps
Jerome himself) would be consciously aware.

Thus we find that Jerome is inhibited in the very
matter in which he is most stimulated. Both his
inhibitions and his desires are concentrated at the
genital level. We shall naturally be inclined to imagine
that causal relations are involved here—relations that
are probably of a circular order. On the one hand,
the inhibitions are probably directed to the sexual act
because the genital desires are so intense; on the other
hand, it may well be that the frustration of end-pleasure
that is thus brought about by damming up the natural
channel of discharge (and thus maintaining libidinal

tension at a high level) produces an obsessive preoccupation with fore-pleasure that is responsible for Jerome's striking continuity of sexual interests (No. 5).

In No. 9 (degree of sex differentiation) we seem to see a consequence of several of the preceding items. A high degree of differentiation between the sexes goes naturally with complexity and sophistication rather than with simplicity and naïveté (Nos. 1 and 2). It is a characteristic of adult life rather than of childhood (No. 3). In so far as it manifests itself in gallantry and chivalry on the part of the man, in coyness and coquetry on the part of the woman (which are the sex distinctions that here come chiefly into consideration), it is a difference that is in harmony with a romantic rather than a matter-of-fact outlook or tradition (No. 4). It obviously implies a preoccupation with the specifically sexual aspects of life rather than with the general interests that are common to both sexes (No. 5); it implies too at least a fairly high degree of genital supremacy (No. 6), higher at any rate than that involved in Uni's love of pugilism. Matters are more complex and less obvious as regards Nos. 7 and 8, but, on the whole, sex differentiation of the kind here in question seems undoubtedly to involve something of the subtle interplay of desire and inhibition that we discussed under these heads. Both gallantry and coquetry imply an inhibition at the more direct and unsublimated levels, and a dallying at, and accentuaion of, the stage of fore-pleasure. In fact, they are among the most obvious, but also most remarkable, examples of the prolongation, complication and intensification of desire through inhibition that are to be met with in human life— examples that are the more interesting in that they are not confined to human life, but, in the phenomena of courtship, are to be seen, at least in rudimentary form, in many species of animals.

There seems no doubt that the contrast in this matter between Jerome and Uni is really to some extent characteristic of the cultures which they represent. The Latin countries are the true homes of gallantry and of flirtation, whereas the northern countries have been the chief centres of the feminist movements, which have aimed (to a considerable extent successfully) at the reduction of sex differences, alike in love and life. Chivalry and coquettishness have both a certain fundamental incompatibility with equality of the sexes in work and in play, in politics and marriage. In France there has been but little demand for women's suffrage, women being on the whole content with a certain compensating privilege and glamour with which their very sex endowed them. In Norway, on the other hand, stress has been laid on the common features which women share with men, and little value has been placed upon forms of politeness and of gallantry that have seemed to northern eyes to be, at best, superfluous, and, at worst, hypocritical, degrading and insulting.

The desire for secrecy and intrigue (No. 10), clearly depends to some extent upon a projection of intrapsychic conflicts. Just as, in Jerome's individual mind, desires lose their spice and piquancy unless accompanied by inhibitions, so in his social and sexual life, actions tend to become pointless except so far as they involve the overcoming of dangers and obstacles, the fear of which affords a justification for secrecy, deception and roundabout procedure. Here again there are cultural differences corresponding to the mental differences between the protagonists of Bedel's book. Latin culture and the Latin languages are riddled with courteous minor hypocrisies and insincerities, which are neglected, despised or actively condemned in the majority of northern countries, in which a blunter and more direct form of speech is preferred. It is Latin culture too which affords the most fruitful ground for intrigue and that subtle art of putting a soft gloss on hard and stubborn attitudes that is called diplomacy. Even such minor forms of economic subtlety and indirectness as are involved in bargaining have their European home in Latin countries, whereas the more direct and matter-of-fact system of fixed prices makes greater appeal to the northerner, anxious to get his business done as expeditiously, and with as little fuss, as possible.

Very similar factors play a part in No. 11 (amount of agreement between theory and practice). The need for obstacles to the satisfaction of libido can very conveniently and profitably avail itself of the impedi ments to desire afforded by conventional morality. While partial (or at any rate nominal) adherence to the dictates of this morality satisfies the super-ego, trans- gression of these dictates adds a pleasant piquancy to the gratification of desire. Hence in Jerome's type both aspects of the mind are contented with existing social conventions, and there is little desire to bridge the gap that separates them from individual practice. To the simpler mentality of the Uni type, however, such a gap is much less easily tolerated, so that there results a constant endeavour to bring ethical theory and individual practice into harmony with one another; with the result that social and legal sanctions become less severe, though adherence to them is at the same time much more rigid. Here again there are cultural parallels. In the attempt to achieve the harmony in question, several northern nations have made fairly drastic reductions in the oppressiveness of the social and legal institutions corresponding to the super-ego, while on the other hand there would seem to be a more sincere and honest endeavour to live up to these institutions as they actually exist. To take just one example of this difference—Roman Catholic countries seem to tolerate easily the simultaneous existence of a theoretically monogamous and indissoluble marriage with the widespread practice of extramarital intercourse, while in the countries of which Uni is a representative there tends to be on the one hand less rigidity in the marriage laws but, on the other hand, considerably less enjoyment of sexual freedom outside marriage or at any rate betrothal (as is shown for instance by the very much smaller illegitimate birth-rate that is characteristic of these latter countries). And I believe that examination would show that what is true of the marriage laws is true of the great majority of other laws. The French have (according at least to reputation) a habit—one that has proved very irritating to co-operating foreign governments—of meeting many abuses by the simple maxim "*affichez*"—a maxim which eases the conscience and leaves practice largely where it was

On the other hand the greater necessity of really conforming to official institutions that is found in the North may sometimes lead to a greater fear of making these institutions too clear-cut or definite. This may be an important factor, for instance, in the English tendency to "muddle through" rather than to rely on detailed plans or principles. The English constitution and legal system have grown up out of a thousand *ad hoc* adjustments and decisions. There is a fear of logic that is foreign to the Latin mind, perhaps because the Anglo-

Saxon can less easily tolerate a departure from logical principles when once established. It may be the fear thus engendered that is responsible for the charge of hypocrisy that the French sometimes level against the English—a charge that is apt to seem unjustified to the English themselves, because they are unable to tolerate the mental conflicts concerned and hence fail to recognize their existence.

Much the same general considerations apply again to No. 12 (attitude to conventional propriety), except that here the ethical sanctions that satisfy the inhibitions (and through this stimulate the libido) are much less projected and externalized as institutions, but are more purely psychic—albeit psychic possessions of the group, and not merely of the individual. Jerome and his compeers are prepared to pay their respects to the convention that there shall be no sexual intercourse until after marriage, though they do not seriously intend that their own actions shall conform to this convention. Uni and those of her persuasion substitute a more "advanced" convention of their own, so that theory and practice may, here again, be harmonized. Far from deriving an added pleasure from a discrepancy between the demands of the social super-ego and the claims of instinct, such people experience an urgent need to establish a recognized and fully conscious compromise between the two. With them everything must be—to use two favourite phrases—"in order" and "above board"—a condition which to Jerome's type of mind deprives libidinal satisfaction of a great deal of its value. Jerome's philosophy in this matter (which would be the very opposite of Uni's, if she had one) could not be better expressed than in words that Mr. Aldous Huxley puts into the mouth of one of his characters: "Emancipation is excellent, no doubt, in its way. But in the end it defeats its own object. People ask for freedom, but what they finally get turns out to be boredom. To those for whom love has become as obvious an affair as eating dinner, for whom there are no blushful mysteries, no reticences, no fancy-fostering concealment, but only plain speaking and the facts of nature—how flat and stale the whole business must become! It needs crinolines to excite the imagination and dragonish duennas to inflame desire to passion."

Psychology is still woefully ignorant about the fascinating problem of the overestimation of the sexual object that is involved in romantic love (No. 13). But from psycho-analytic work, especially that of Freud himself, three things at least are fairly clear about the process of "falling in love:" (a) that it demands some inhibition of the more immediate and direct sexual desires (it is to this extent "aim-inhibited"), (b) that the lover tends to see in his beloved the image of some previously loved person, (c) that the super-ego is projected on to the beloved and is then seized upon as an object by the libido, to the impoverishment of the ego itself. In the case of (a) and (c) at least, we can discern factors with which we are familiar in the psychology of Jerome. We have already seen that his libido is to some extent "aim-inhibited"—at least as regards the final aim of sex. His super-ego, too, is in certain respects more highly developed and exigent than is that of Uni. It is perhaps not surprising then that, if projected, it can seem an object worthy of a worship to which a projection of Uni's more modest super-ego could scarcely claim. Here we see in another form the advantage which the libido can derive from a stern super-ego. The imagined perfections of a beloved person can probably only exist in so far as they represent the projection of a similarly "perfect" super-ego—and a super-ego such as Uni's, that has struck an open bargain with the instincts can no longer be perfect in this sense.

The tendency indicated under heading (b) clearly depends upon some degree of fixation on the parent or other early love object, a fixation that in turn probably depends upon an inhibition of such genital impulses as are necessary for the due displacement of infantile incestuous affection. Here again, then, inhibition favours "falling in love." There is of course too a subtle interaction between (b) and (c), inasmuch as the loved parent furnishes some of the constituents of the super-ego that is projected on to the person with whom one falls in love.[1] The fact that Jerome, like other members of the Don Juan type, can find no permanent satisfaction in any one love object is probably due in part to the fact that no woman can in reality "live up" to the perfections either of the mother-*imago* or of the projected portion of the super-ego, partly to the fear of losing the romantic element of overestimation once the inhibitions have been overcome (a fear which Jerome frequently expresses), partly to the workings of the still persisting incest inhibition (which is responsible for the actual impotence or sexual disability), and partly to an obsessive need for reassurance against the effects of this latter disability, a need which constantly seeks

___

[1] It is probable that we have to do here with the kinder, more loving and more lovable aspects of the super-ego, at the existence of which Freud has hinted, for instance, in his recent paper on Humour (*International Journal of Psycho-analysis*, 1928, IX, 1). But a discussion of this would take us too far afield. Altogether, there is urgent need for the further study of the problems involved in falling in love, with especial reference to the rôle of the parent *imago* and the super-ego.

K

for fresh signs of the capacity to make sexual conquests. In any case the existence of a mother-fixation in Jerome is indicated by a long and apologetic letter which he writes to his mother, announcing (but not till the fourth page) his engagement to Uni and asking for her benediction and approval, without which he felt himself unable to make any permanent decision.

That the tendency of the Jerome type to jealousy (No. 14) is connected with several of the previous items, especially with the last four, is sufficiently obvious. Secrecy, intrigue, suspicion, the clandestine overstepping of legal ties or conventional restrictions form an atmosphere in which jealousy can flourish, whereas frankness, "advanced" moral notions and an absence of the intenser forms of overestimation of the love object are all unfavourable to jealousy. The desire for obstacles which is so essential to Jerome makes a rival almost a necessary part of the total picture of his love affairs, which only the utter absence of all opposition keeps in the background during the greater part of Bedel's story. Psycho-analytic theory has shown, moreover, that jealousy is largely dependent upon unconscious factors, *e.g.* the persistence of an Œdipus attitude and, above all, a homosexually determined identification with the loved person whose infidelity is feared—factors that imply fixations and correlative inhibitions that have prevented the free development of the libido. It is the complicated path that the libido has been compelled to take that is responsible for the ready liability to jealousy, as for so many other features in the Jerome mentality. Here again, too, Jerome is typical of his country; for France is a land in which jealousy is not only condoned, but to some extent approved and even admired, as is shown by its traditional attitude towards the *crime passionnel*.

After all that has been said, there is no need to stress the fact that Jerome's character is essentially neurotic (No. 15), depending as it does for its intimate make-up upon a subtle compromise between libido and inhibition, of a kind that is thoroughly characteristic of neurosis. Uni's mind, on the other hand, appears to be free of the conflicts that we regard as neurotic, though at the same time, as already noted, it strikes us as more primitive and childish.

III

THE UNDERLYING PRINCIPLE AND ITS APPLICATIONS

Summarizing the differences in the two types before us, we find that one big factor—that depending upon the interaction of inhibition and libido—accounts for, or at least plays a part in, nearly all the 15 distinctions that we have enumerated. In Jerome the libido has adapted itself to the presence of inhibitions, and has, as it were, struck such a satisfactory compromise with them that it is wellnigh incapable of functioning in their absence—all the zest of life is dependent upon obstacles or inhibitions of one kind or another. In Uni on the other hand, there has been no such compromise. Her super-ego has been in certain respects more moderate in its demands, but at the same time sterner in the insistence on those which it has made, and less corruptible in the face of temptations to commute for them in terms of suffering. Her libido has therefore had to accustom itself to obtaining satisfaction without the extra spice of overcoming inhibitions. Her super-ego and libido have to make their peace in a more direct

fashion, without the formation of those subtle com-
promises that satisfy the one while at the same time
increasing (in certain spheres and within certain limits
at least) the gratification of the other.   Hence the
generally simpler and more naïve pattern of her mind.

It is clear that the mental difference between our
two types raises several interesting problems of psychological economics and dynamics.   There is for instance
the problem of determining more precisely the rôles
of the super-ego and the libido in the compromise that
is arrived at.

We said just now that Uni's super-ego was in certain
respects more moderate in its demands.   Uni is in a
certain sense more "advanced" and freer in her outlook and her actions.   But this greater freedom is only
obtained at the price of a greater obedience.   To Uni,
conflict between libido and the super-ego is intolerable;
hence her actions must always be capable of moral
justification.   Jerome is much more tolerant of guilt.
This is of course a condition of his capacity for moral
compromise.   His conflicts are nearer the surface, and
he would therefore make an easier subject for analysis.
Uni's repressions would seem to have taken place at a
deeper level.   It is this perhaps that makes her super-
ego less "corruptible."   We get the impression that
Uni's attitude represents a method of solving conflicts
that is characteristic of the puritanical mind.   Her
super-ego has retained its severity but has become
"enlightened."   If she had not been an "advanced"
young lady, she might have been a Fundamentalist.
But we have to recognize that it is on the basis of such a
solution that the moral progress of the Western world
has been made.   The solution in terms of compromise
that is characteristic of the Jerome type does not make

for rapid moral change; both super-ego and libido are too satisfied with the bargains they have struck.

As regards Jerome's mentality, there is the further problem as to how far we are really justified in speaking with Alexander of the "corruptibility" of the super-ego, and in what way and to what extent the method of corruption, *i.e.*, the endurance of pain, provides satisfaction both to the super-ego and to the masochistic components of the libido. With regard to the libido, there is the fascinating problem of how far the increased gratification that the libido eventually obtains from the very existence of inhibitions can be described in quantitative terms, how far only in terms of qualitative differences. The earliest psycho-analytic discovery of an example of this general mechanism—that concerning the child's tendency to postpone defæcation in order to enjoy greater eventual pleasure from the act —suggests something in the nature of a simple quantitative increase in tension. But there are many other manifestations of the same principle—including most of those with which we have been concerned—which seem, superficially at any rate, to be describable only in qualitative terms; the words "piquant" (note the implication of pain) and—in German—"*raffiniert*" inevitably suggest themselves in this connection. If there are both qualitative and quantitative factors at work, can the quantitative factors be described as simply due to increase of tension without change of channel, while the qualitative factors correspond to (partial or complete) displacements? There is a further problem as to the relation of the main *principle of increase of satisfaction through inhibition* (as we may perhaps designate it) to the degree of genital supremacy in the structure of the libido. The data we have examined reveal a positive correspondence between the use made of this principle and the degree of such supremacy— but we were not able to show with any assurance in what way one factor depended on the other.

This problem leads to the still more general one of how far a gradual increase in the use of the principle is to be regarded as a normal feature of development. On the one hand it may seem an essential element of culture, yet on the other hand it has the closest relationship to mechanisms that we have learnt to look upon as characteristically neurotic. If we knew with more certainty what differentiates the neurotic from the healthy in this matter, we should have achieved a considerable gain in psychopathological insight and at the same time have made a distinct forward step in the application of psychology to ethical, educational and sociological problems.

Here, however, we must be content to indicate these questions without attempting to answer them. We may, however, in conclusion, be allowed a few words concerning some of the very numerous and diverse phenomena in which the principle we have been discussing would seem to play a part. Such a review— even of the briefest and most fragmentary kind—will at least serve to convince us of the very wide application and great importance of the principle and will perhaps enable us to arrive at some provisional conclusion as regards its general function and value in the process of mental development.

Let us start with instances of a purely sensory kind. We have already mentioned the early discovery by psycho-analysis of the application of the principle in the anal sphere; a similar mechanism can sometimes be observed in the case of urethral erotism, for retention of the urine can undoubtedly lead to greater pleasure in eventual micturition. More complicated, however, are the manifestations of the principle in the case of oral erotism. Not only do hunger and thirst add greatly to the enjoyment of eating and drinking, but we often derive an increased pleasure from food and drink that contain an element that by itself is unpleasant. Indeed, the word "piquant," which I have found myself led to use on more than one occasion, is a term that is often employed with special reference to the pleasures of taste. Some palates have lost the taste for simple food and have to be tempted with pungent, sour or bitter ingredients that seem disagreeable to less sophisticated tastes—much as Jerome has no taste for sexual adventure unless it contains elements of the forbidden, the intriguing and the dangerous, which are pointless or repellent to the simpler mind of Uni. A further aspect of the principle in the oral sphere concerns the very method and manner of eating and drinking. The glutton may bolt his food in a few moments like a dog, whereas the epicure delays the complete gratification of his hunger, commencing his meal with dainty *hors d'oeuvres* that stimulate rather than satisfy, prolonging his repast so as to get the maximum of satisfaction from it and preserving some of the daintiest morsels till the end (a form of temporary renunciation that is shown even by the human infant, but not by the dog).

Similar considerations apply to the genital sphere, where the epicure will prolong the sexual act, though the postponement of orgasm may involve control and renunciation of the most intense kind. Here, indeed, more perhaps than anywhere else, is to be seen the most intimate and exquisite combination of inhibition and desire, frustration and satisfaction proceeding by parallel and equal steps, the former being clearly and inevitably a condition of the latter. In the activity of the masochistic elements, moreover, we see the classic instance of the fusion of moral and instinctual factors to which Freud drew attention in his pioneering attack on the subtle problems presented by this component of the sexual impulse.

Leaving the sensory level for a wider field, we find our principle at work throughout the complicated procedures that lead up to the sexual act. Indeed a great deal of fore-pleasure is directly due to its operation, and, as we have already indicated, both the sexual play of coquetry and the more exalted and emotionalized phenomena of romantic love seem to depend to a large extent upon it—being in the nature of an efflorescence of libido occurring as a result of the inhibition of more primitive forms of gratification.

Another field where the principle operates is that of humour, which, as Freud has also shown, is a form of satisfaction that results from a certain method of overcoming inhibitions, and which could not exist without these inhibitions. The "smutty" joke, for instance, gives pleasure just because it infringes a sexual taboo, and can be fully appreciated only where the inhibiting and instinctual forces are present in the right proportion (and perhaps also in the proper kind of fusion). Too high a degree of freedom or repression is apt to make such jokes seem either pointless or disgusting.

The "smutty" joke constitutes perhaps but one particular example of the general attraction that is exercised by the forbidden. For an action to be forbidden may give that action a relish which it would not otherwise possess. Here, however, our principle is complicated by the operation of revolutionary tendencies (springing probably in the last resort from the Œdipus complex) into which we cannot enter here.

Not so different from the "smutty" joke as might at first appear is the pleasure derived from talking scandal and generally dilating on the infringements of sexual taboos by other people—a form of enjoyment that has its childish counterpart in the delight that many children have in hearing of the misdeeds of very "naughty" children or inventing such misdeeds in the case of dolls or imaginary companions. The chief psychical difference between these cases and the smutty joke is that the rôle of the libidinal element is here less clearly recognized, since it is projected on to the transgressors—a mechanism which makes libidinal satisfaction compatible with the simultaneous enjoyment of a pharisaical self-righteousness. At one stage further in the effort towards rationalization we get the purity campaign. Here the super-ego has definitely entered into an alliance with the sadistic elements of the libido, and libidinal satisfaction is derived, not only from the contemplation but the persecution of those who have indulged in the forbidden pleasures.

Many striking manifestations of our principle are to be seen in the sphere of modesty and dress. Clothes, which impede the more primitive manifestations both of exhibitionism and of scoptophilia, have proved a most potent method of stimulating both tendencies. This fact has long been recognized by all who have devoted a little unprejudiced observation to the matter; but in recent years it has been corroborated on a large scale by the practice of nude culture in Germany and other countries, which has made it abundantly manifest that the sacrifice involved in nudity is not so much one of modesty as of an added zest and strength of certain libidinal desires. In fact, clothes are among the most effective aphrodisiacs that have ever been discovered. But this is a subject on which I need not enlarge, as I have elsewhere already treated it in detail.[1]

Dress can indeed be regarded from many points of view as one of the unnecessary luxuries of life— one that, if the upholders of the "simple life" and "back to nature" movements had their way, would be abolished, or at any rate reduced to a bare minimum. And this is calculated to make us realize that many (or perhaps indeed all) luxuries owe something to our principle. For do they not come into existence largely as substitute gratifications for more primitive pleasures that are inhibited? To take just one glaring example. The modern dance hall, with all its complicated paraphernalia of evening dresses, polished dancing floor, coloured lights, jazz band and cocktail bar, is an elaborate and roundabout method of obtaining, in a displaced but still recognizable form, the pleasures of a sexual orgy—pleasures that might be obtained in an infinitely simpler way, if our cultural restrictions and inhibitions had not rendered the simpler and more direct gratification impossible.

And here we embark on a few final reflections and evaluations of the principle we have been studying. Of what value is the principle to culture and in what ways is it superfluous and pathological? It would seem that we have come up here against the old problem of the distinction between sublimation and neurosis. It is a problem that can scarcely receive a final solution without touching upon intricate and disputable points of ethical theory. But here, as elsewhere, a provisional hedonistic criterion may be adopted by saying that the

---

[1] *The Psychology of Clothes.* London : Hogarth Press. 1930.

ultimate aim of sublimation, and indeed of all mental development, should be the attainment of the maximum of pleasure in accordance with the reality principle.

According to this standard we should recognize that the ability to tolerate the pain of temporary inhibition is a very necessary condition of progress, and we should welcome the fact that this inhibition may under certain circumstances lead to an increase of eventual satisfaction, since it seems a providential arrangement of nature to compensate for the discomfort and anxiety inevitably caused by frustration. Indeed, as I ventured to point out some thirteen years ago,[1] this fact to some extent affects the pessimistic considerations of Freud with regard to the sacrifices of enjoyment that culture has demanded. But, nevertheless, we must go on to ask two questions: (a) how far are the inhibitions really necessary, i.e. imposed by the reality principle? (b) how far does any increase of satisfaction that results from the inhibition really compensate for the loss? If the inhibitions are essential for ulterior reasons, i.e. in order to achieve some eventual greater pleasure of another kind or to avoid some eventual greater pain, we must submit to them, even though there is no adequate compensation in terms of added strength or piquancy of the desires that are inhibited. But if this is not the case, then we may apply the hedonistic criterion to the narrower sphere of these desires themselves, and ask, do we, in respect of the eventual satisfaction of these desires, gain or lose by the inhibition? An actual hedonistic calculus is not easy to apply. As regards some simpler forms of inhibition, however, there

---

[1] In a paper on " The Biological Basis of Sexual Repression and its Sociological Significance, *British Journal of Psychology* (*Medical Section*), 1921, I, p. 251.

seems little doubt that the gain is greater than the loss
—as, for instance, in the prolongation and refinement
of sensory pleasure in eating and drinking and the
sexual act. Most people would agree too that the same
applies to many forms of sexual fore-pleasure, such as
those involved in flirting. But when it comes to the
more complicated manifestations of our principle, such
as the pleasures of intrigue and secrecy, the attraction
of the forbidden, the maintenance for hedonistic reasons
of clearly out-of-date social and ethical conventions,
the demand for the more elaborate and extravagant
forms of luxury, we shall begin to have serious doubts.

In view of the difficulty of an actual hedonistic
calculus, we may resort to two substitutive criteria of a
qualitative kind. (1) Approaching the matter from the
point of view of the super-ego, we may ask if there is
present some element of guilt that has to be atoned for
by suffering. If so, there is a presumption that the
suffering is unnecessary and fulfils no useful purpose.
From our psycho-analytical knowledge we should be
inclined to say that there is a strong element of such
unnecessary suffering in the majority of individual compulsions and obsessions and in their social equivalents,
ritual and ceremonial—in most of which pain, boredom
or irritation predominate over pleasure. Here again,
however, there may be some compulsions of the simpler
sort that bring more pleasure than pain and in which
asceticism seems to have acquired a definitely epicurean
tinge—as in the case of the man who had himself
awakened regularly two hours before it was actually time
to get up, in order that he might consciously realize the
luxury of bed, or in the case of another who sometimes
got out of a warm bath for a few moments in order to re-
experience the joy of entering it, enhanced by the contrast

it presented to the relatively chilly air. (2) Approaching
the matter this time from the side of the libido, we may
ask whether the satisfactions of the libido have become
so dependent on the presence of inhibitions that there is
incapacity for satisfaction without them—as for instance
in the inability to enjoy the pleasures of sex without the
element of the forbidden. If so, there is surely an unnecessary sacrifice of the possibility of simpler and, as
we say, more "natural" pleasures, indicating that,
quite apart from ulterior consequences (which are not
always of the desirable variety), the possibility of the
more exotic and refined pleasures has been bought at
too heavy a cost. As a general rule, education and
development should be such as to permit of more
complex pleasures without losing the capacity to enjoy
the simpler ones, and although this may not everywhere be possible, we may say that the demand for
such a condition as, for instance, an obstacle to be
overcome or a convention to be flouted, before sexual
pleasures can be enjoyed, indicates a neurotic element
which is a hindrance rather than a help to ethical
progress.

We suspect that the price that has been paid in these
cases is that which has been necessary to "corrupt"
the super-ego. It is indeed in the alliance between the
super-ego and the libido that we have to seek the
intimate workings of the mechanism that we have been
studying. A closer determination of the economic
and dynamic aspects of this alliance is beyond doubt
one of the most important tasks for psycho-analytic
research in the immediate future.

In this paper I have touched but lightly on a subject
which upon examination opens up somewhat discon-
certingly until, in its ultimate ramifications, it appears

to embrace almost the whole length and breadth of human culture ·As such it is a subject that requires for its elucidation a volume rather than a single paper —a volume, however, that can only be written in the future, as the result of much further detailed psychological investigation. What I have here written, will, I hope, be looked upon indulgently as the first, and quite provisional, reflections of a psychologist upon the problem presented by M. Bedel in so fascinating and challenging a fashion.

ESPERANTO AND THE INTERNATIONAL LANGUAGE MOVEMENT.[1]

I

ESPERANTO AND ITS FOUNDER

It is now fifty years since the movement in favour of the adoption of an international auxiliary language came before the cultured Western world as a serious practical proposition. The idea of such a language dates back to a much earlier period, Descartes and Leibnitz being among the first and most illustrious who have concerned themselves with the question. But it was the first congress of Volapükists at Friedrichshafen in 1884 that definitely marked the emergence of

---

[1] Reprinted from *The International Journal of Psycho-analysis*, Vol. **VI**, 1925, Part II.

an international language from the study of the philo-
sopher or philologist into the practical affairs of everyday life.   Since that time, although the movement
itself has had a chequered history, the majority of
cultured individuals in the more progressive countries
have been vaguely aware of the possibility of international language, and dimly conscious of its desirability
on general grounds, while there has been a continual stream of enthusiastic individuals engaged in the
elaboration or study of new linguistic schemes or in
the propaganda of some already existing language.
Although the number of those who have in one of these
two ways come closely into touch with the problems
involved is still comparatively small, it is pretty generally recognized, among those competent to judge, that
these problems have some very real importance for the
modern world.   The few congresses of Volapük at
the beginning of this active period, and of Ido in
recent times, together with the far more numerous and
larger congresses of Esperanto that have been held in
many parts of the world during the last thirty years,
have, moreover, shown conclusively that an international language is a perfectly practical proposition
from the linguistic point of view.   A study of the
psychological factors underlying or connected with
this movement in favour of an international language
should, therefore, have some interest for the social
psychologist and sociologist, especially as such a study
promises to throw some additional light on two general
fields of outstanding interest, the psychology of progressive social movements and the psychology of
language.   The present communication does not aspire
to do more than to afford an introduction to such a
study, based for the most part on the writer's personal

association with the Esperanto movement for a considerable number of years.

One of the most immediately striking aspects of the Esperanto movement, an aspect which often proves astonishing, and sometimes disconcerting, to those who happen to come across any considerable body of Esperantists without previous acquaintance with the movement, is its enthusiastic and quasi-religious character. It soon becomes apparent that, with the majority of Esperantists, it is not so much the language in and for itself, as a simple medium of communication, that inspires their devotion. It is rather the so-called "internal idea" of Esperantism (the aim of international and inter-racial fraternity based on mutual understanding and sympathy) that underlies the purely linguistic features of the movement, and causes the language itself to be looked upon as an instrument or as a symbol rather than as an end in itself; a symbol however which, like other symbols, has itself acquired a high emotional value ("la kara lingvo") through its association with the ultimate aim for which it stands.

It is in this respect that the history of Esperanto would seem to differ most markedly from the history of its less successful competitors. It is a respect in which the history of the language has, through the feelings and activities of its adherents, mirrored the thoughts and aspirations of its inventor. For Zamenhof the language, however great the pains he bestowed upon it, was never more than a stepping-stone to the higher goal of human love that should transcend the barriers of language, race and nationality. The remarkable personality of the founder of Esperanto is indeed, beyond all doubt, to a very large extent responsible

L

both for the character of the Esperanto movement and for the relatively large amount of success which it has hitherto enjoyed. Zamenhof's peculiar combination of personal modesty, high idealism, linguistic ability, scientific empiricism, and keen foresight in practical affairs, enabled him not only to give to the world an artificial language which was, by general admission, greatly superior to anything that had hitherto been devised, but also to inspire in his followers a very high degree of admiration and devotion for his own person, his philanthropic ideals and his linguistic creation. In the minds of many thousands of Esperantists he has stood for the ideal father, a father characterized at once by loving kindness and creative power. His love, in particular, was of such a kind as to realize to an unusual extent the fiction which, according to Freud,[1] tends to underlie all organized groups of human beings, viz. that the leader (father *imago*) loves all his followers (children) equally. For was not Zamenhof's gift to the world one that was of value to *all* humanity without distinction?[2] At the same time, by his renunciation of all special ownership, privilege or control with regard to Esperanto (a matter in which his attitude differed markedly from that of some other inventors of languages, notably Schleyer and de Beaufront, the authors of Volapük and Ido respectively), he tended to prevent the transference to himself of the more hostile aspects of the father *imago*; only those Esper-antists who were exceptionally sensitive in the matter of paternal authority, or whose ideals differed very

---

[1] *Group Psychology and Analysis of the Ego*, p. 42.

[2] Perhaps, too, there is an echo of the same idea in Zamenhof's own contention that " every country belongs equally—in the material and in the moral sense—to all its children." " Letero al Diplomatio," published in various Esperanto journals early in 1915.

markedly from Zamenhof's,[1] could be alienated from Esperanto through disagreement with its founder.

While this renunciation of power was undoubtedly advantageous in reducing the displacement of father-regarding hostility on general grounds, it may very well be that the other aspect of the Œdipus complex also played a part in very many cases. Patriotic feelings for one's native land are, we know, very frequently derived in part from displacement of the mother-regarding affects; our native land is our mother. Such patriotic feelings, moreover, frequently pass over to the language of our native land; patriotic outbursts often have, not only their political, but their linguistic side; as when a struggle for political independence on the part of any given people goes hand in hand with a revival of what is affectionately termed the mother-tongue, *Muttersprache* [2] (the same connection being manifested when a superior power endeavours to stamp out the nationality of a smaller people by abolishing its political independence, and at the same time prohibiting or discouraging its language.) Associations similarly derived from the mother are probably operative to some extent in the case of Esperanto. If this is so, it is clear that Zamenhof's abandonment of all special ownership of the language constitutes an important symbolic wish fulfilment in relation to the Œdipus complex. It is true that the fundamental wish underlying this complex is only half fulfilled; even if

---

[1] Though he constantly endeavoured to placate these latter by his repeated insistence (from the " Boulogne Declaration " of 1905 onwards) that the use or propaganda of Esperanto did not necessarily imply allegiance to his own or any other political and social ideals, such ideals being a purely private matter in his own case, and in that of all other Esperantists.

[2] Whereas the term " father-tongue," corresponding to " father-land," does not occur, at least in any language with which I am familiar.

the father abandons his special claims upon the mother, there remains the incest taboo between son and mother, though this taboo becomes more bearable when sons and father are on an equal footing. Some indications of the presence of this taboo may perhaps be found in the stringent rule relating to the *netuŝebleco*, the inviolability, of the "*Fundamento.*"[1] With the consent and approval of his early followers, Zamenhof himself, although abandoning every other claim to control the language, laid it down that, whatever might be the evolution of the language in other respects, there should be no tampering with this *Fundamento*, adherence to which should be absolutely obligatory to every Esperantist—an obligation that has been strictly adhered to by all who have remained within the Esperanto camp, but which, significantly enough, has been regarded as an intolerable restriction by those who have gone over to Ido or to other schemes (in all probability those in whom the love attitude towards Zamenhof was not sufficiently powerful to bring about a willing acquiescence in the incest barrier in its displaced form as relating to the language).

Whatever degree of truth there may be in this suggestion that the language itself has in certain respects become the object of a displacement of the mother-regarding tendencies, there can be little doubt that the Esperanto movement has enjoyed a very fortunate disposition of those aspects of the Œdipus complex that relate to the father, and it is probable that the relatively large success of Esperanto is to a considerable extent due to this fact. The whole attitude of Zamenhof has been such as to foster love, loyalty and respect towards him as a father-substitute and friendliness towards fellow-men

---

[1] *I.e.* the fundamental rules of grammar and vocabulary.

as brothers whom the father favours with an equal love. What father-hatred inevitably persists is displaced on to vague and impersonal figures representing chauvinist or tyrannical governmental authorities, figures which are for the most part too indefinite to permit of the development of well-marked sentiments of hate. For the rest, Esperantists are looked upon as constituting one large family circle (*unu granda rondo familia*, in the words of the Esperanto hymn, *La Espero*), a circle which it is the object of all ardent propagandists continually to widen until it includes all the populations of the earth.

II

ESPERANTO AND PRIMITIVE CHRISTIANITY

The Esperanto movement, with its quasi-religious enthusiasm and its attempt to break down the barriers between nations and races, inevitably challenges comparison with certain other movements of a universalizing tendency. It has, of course, certain features in common with Socialism and Communism. These also are international and pacifist in character, and aim at fostering a spirit of comradeship among fellow-members; but they differ from the Esperanto movement in two important respects:

(*a*) In the essential economic basis of their programme;

(*b*) In that the revolutionary and insurgent tendencies —based ultimately on displacements of father-hatred—are very much more prominent.

In the Esperanto movement these latter tendencies are implicit rather than explicit, a respect in which, as in several other points, there is—if the comparison be allowed—a marked resemblance to the Christian religion in its early stages. Indeed, to one who has been in close touch with the fraternizing and propagandist aspects of the Esperanto movement, it will be fairly clear that this movement has much in common with primitive Christianity. In both cases there is an almost exclusive predominance of the loving attitude towards the father (as distinguished, for instance, from the fear attitude which plays a considerable part in the Jewish religion), a tendency to regard all mankind as brothers (as contrasted with the sharp distinction drawn in some religious and social movements between true believers and outsiders), and a very strong bond of kindness and sympathy between all those who take part in the movement. (Esperantists are, as the present writer can testify from his own experience, extraordinarily kindly and helpful towards one another.) A further important point of resemblance lies in the fact that both primitive Christianity and Esperanto appealed chiefly, not to those possessed of wealth, power, high social standing, or exceptional intelligence, but to the relatively poor, uninfluential, and uncultured. This fact has strongly impressed itself on impersonal outside observers, for in the circular of the Committee on International Auxiliary Language appointed in 1919 by the International Research Council, we read:

"From a sociological standpoint one of the most important features of the whole subject of international language development is the surprising interest and fidelity to the cause shown by the proletariat. It has really been from this class that there has come to the movement not only the great bulk of personal effort, but of financial support as well. It has been truly the multiplication of the "widow's mite" which has supported the work thus far. This is strongly reflected, for example, in both the texts and the clientèle of the approximately one hundred journals which were being published in Esperanto alone at the outbreak of the war."[1]

This predominantly proletarian support is an interesting phenomenon, which is of course common to many progressive movements besides primitive Christianity and Esperanto, and it would take us too far afield to go into its general causes here. We shall, however, have occasion to refer later on to certain particular factors of importance in the case of Esperanto (p. 201). Meanwhile, we need only note the fact that this proletarian support often results in a certain crudity of manner, both as regards the expressions of loyalty within the movement and the methods of propaganda employed in relation to the outer world—a crudity which is apt to react unfavourably upon cultured persons who are otherwise in sympathy with the movement. There is little doubt but that a similar tendency to crudeness must have characterized many of the activities of the early Christians and produced a very similar prejudice in the mind of many a cultured Greek and Roman.

Another feature which the Esperanto movement has in common with Christianity is the saintlike nature of its founder. Some of the foremost features of Zamenhof's character are peculiarly reminiscent of the personality of Christ. From very early days, Zamenhof seems to have been imbued with a sense of responsibility for the welfare of his fellow-men. The fact that

[1] Quoted by Guérard, *A Short History of the International Language Movement*, p. 185 ; see also Privat, *Vivo de Zamenhof*, p. 86.

inter-racial discord and want of mutual understanding between those who spoke different languages appeared to him to be the supreme evils that beset humanity was due largely to the circumstances of his early life in the little town of Bialistock, on what was then the border between West Russia and Russian Poland; for in that part of Central Europe the need for inter-racial sympathy and understanding, and for some common tongue as a means of such understanding, is much more acutely perceptible than in most other parts of the civilized world. But that he was so powerfully affected by the evident miseries due to racial antagonisms must be set down to a natural sympathy with the sufferings of others, a sympathy either inherited from his mother or implanted by her influence and teaching. For it was from her that he appears to have derived the principal characteristics of his affective life, his devotion to and absorption in the happiness of others, his remarkable absence of selfishness or desire for mastery, his patience, charity and toleration;[1] while from his father he acquired his more intellectual attributes, linguistic ability, and practical insight, together with his sense of duty and perseverance in an enterprise once undertaken. It was from his mother, too, that he acquired the doctrine that all men were equal before God. His mother, however, unlike his father, belonged to the Jewish religion as well as to the Jewish race. In his early boyhood, doubtless under maternal influence, Zamenhof also was a believer, but ceased

[1] " He never sinned " was a remark of an old servant of his after his death, while even in his early years at school, his biographer tells us, " he constantly avoided causing suffering to anyone," and in later life " he was looked upon by all, by wife, brothers, children, nieces, friends and patients [he was an oculist by profession] as a man of saintly character." Privat, *Vivo de Zamenhof*, pp. 34, 198.

to be so about the time of puberty, and, after passing through a period of severe depression (loss of loved object), eventually attained peace of mind by substituting humanity for God,[1] by placing his trust in that "high moral force which each man carries in his heart" (to quote the words of his speech at the first Esperanto Congress in 1905).

This "high moral force" to be found in all humanity seems very like a fusion of the moral ideas of father and mother respectively. The equality of all humanity in a religious sense was his mother's contribution, while his father "had only one religious faith, namely, the most punctilious devotion to duty."[2]

It may well be that this fusion helped materially in the psychical process of overcoming the primitive hostility towards his father—a process which was carried out with a high degree of success, but which cannot have been altogether easy; both because of the general severity of the father's moral tone (which must have seemed cruel and relentless to the young boy), especially in contrast to the loving kindness of the mother, and because the father was opposed to what he regarded as his son's waste of time and energy upon fanciful linguistic activities (he made the young man promise to abandon these activities for two years, which were to be devoted exclusively to medical studies at Moscow, and then during his absence destroyed the manuscript containing his scheme of international language). Such hostility to the father as was not overcome in this or other ways manifested itself, we may fairly assume, as in the case of the Esperanto movement as a whole, in the effort to defeat the forces of inertia, derision or definite antagonism that were

[1] Privat, *op. cit.*, p. 54.   [2] Privat, *op. cit.*, p. 33.

opposed to the progress of the language and its *interna ideo*. Like many other pacifists, Zamenhof constantly employed the terminology of warfare in reference to his own propaganda, and Esperantists are referred to in their hymn (sung on all occasions on which— *mutatis mutandis*—a national anthem would be appropriate) as *pacaj batalantoj*.

It is in this replacement of God by the moral force of humanity that (apart of course from the mere emphasis on language) there lies perhaps the chief point of difference between the Esperanto movement and early Christianity. But in spite of this difference, it is safe to say that many Esperantists have been dimly aware of a certain similarity between their own movement and the early history of Christianity. It is implied, for instance, in the frequently drawn comparison[1] between Judas, the betrayer of Christ, and de Beaufront, the "betrayer" of Esperanto before the "Delegation for the Adoption of an International Language" in 1906 and 1907.[2] It is implied in the comparison—also fairly frequent—between Esperanto and the Pentecostal gift of tongues to the Apostles; a matter to which we shall refer again. It is implicit

---

[1] Due originally, it would appear, to a remark made by C. Bourlet at the Geneva Congress, 1906. Privat, *op. cit.*, p. 138.

[2] De Beaufront was the official representative of Esperanto at the Delegation, but, in spite of a vigorous opposition to reform proposals shortly before at the second Esperanto Congress, he himself supported Esperanto before the Delegation only on the condition that certain far-reaching reforms should be introduced in accordance with the suggestions contained in an anonymous pamphlet entitled *The Project of Ido*, a pamphlet of which he himself was somewhat later proved to be the author. The history of Ido dates from the publication of this pamphlet and the subsequent adoption of the scheme by the Delegation. For details, see Guérard, *op. cit.*, Chap. VII.

We may note that by Idists, de Beaufront has been called the "St Paul of the Esperanto movement." Cf. L. H. Dyer, *The Problem of an International Auxiliary Language and its Solution in Ido*, p. 63.

perhaps also to some extent in some of Zamenhof's own writings and speeches (*e.g.* in the fine opening paragraphs of his speech before the Boulogne Congress[1]) and may have had some influence on his continual labours in the translation of the Bible, although from the purely practical point of view this was scarcely a necessary or profitable undertaking, since the Bible is beyond doubt already the most widely translated of all extant books, and therefore stands in less need of the assistance of an international language than does any other.

III

ESPERANTO AND OTHER INTERNATIONAL LANGUAGES

As we have seen, the personality of the inventor of Esperanto appears to have made a deep impression on the whole character of the Esperanto movement, this influence being, as we have also seen, very clearly perceptible in the features which differentiate the history of Esperanto from that of most other projects or movements in favour of an international language. These differentiating features, when considered in detail, may perhaps be most conveniently enumerated under four heads:

1. With Zamenhof and the majority of Esperantists, the language, as we have shown, is not so much an end in itself as a means to the higher goal of human fraternity. The whole movement is inspired by a philanthropic—one is tempted to call it a religious—fervour, which is absent in the case of other similar movements. One of the strongest features of Esperanto

---

[1] See Brüggemann, *Historio de Esperanto*, p. 25.

is that it has served as a means of expression for love in a social and sublimated form. The deep arousal of affection that (perhaps in virtue of the mother-identification which we have already considered) is so characteristic of the movement brings it about that the language itself—although logically no more than a means to the desired end—is endowed with far more emotion than are other artificial languages. To the Esperantist the *kara lingvo* is inviolable, beautiful both in itself and in virtue of the great purpose that it serves, and is worthy of being put to the highest literary purposes. Ever since its inception, the more qualified Esperantists have in fact been busy with the translation of the masterpieces of their own native language into Esperanto, with the result that Esperanto is now quite respectably well off from a literary point of view, possessing a list of fine works on all subjects which might well be the envy of many of the smaller national languages.

In the case of the other schemes, the language itself has been the chief object of interest; the whole attitude of the inventor and his followers has been more cognitive and less emotional in nature; above all, there is a lack of the enthusiastic altruism associated with Esperanto. The ultimate concern is with linguistic rather than with social problems. But there is also less delight in the use of the language, less keenness on its propaganda, and on the whole also a more modest attitude with regard to the purposes to which an international language should be applied. Thus many Idists deprecate the activities of Esperantists in the translation of the Classics; in their opinion, the language should be used for everyday purposes of travel, commerce and science, rather than for literary ends.

2. While, in the case of these other schemes, there is less keenness in the *use of* the language, there is obviously more interest in *work on* the language. This leads to the important second distinction, namely, the constant tendency to introduce changes into other languages, as opposed to the attitude of *netuŝebleco* in the case of Esperanto. This difference is important not only from the linguistic and psychological points of view (we have already suggested the nature of its connection with the Œdipus complex), but also from the point of view of practical success. A language which is constantly undergoing modifications imposed by an authority from above is still in the experimental stage (which is the stage that really interests most of the supporters of languages other than Esperanto), and is not likely to be widely used; for only a very few linguistic enthusiasts will take the trouble to learn a language which may undergo vital modifications in a few years' time. Esperanto has remained unchanged, except for natural and inevitable additions to its vocabulary, since its first publication in 1887, and its relatively great success from the point of view of practical adoption has amply justified the conservatism of the Esperantists.

All other movements that have attained any importance have been characterized by change in or of the language selected. Thus Volapük, after a short but brilliant career of about ten years, was wrecked on the question of modifications and improvements (any imperfections in the language itself cannot account for the extreme rapidity of its death). But the Academy which presided over Volapük continued to exist, and passed through a most varied and eventful history. Created at the second Volapük Congress in 1887 under the title of *Kadem bevünetik volapüka*, it gradually "brushed away the *débris* of old Volapük," and in 1903, as the *Akademi de Lingu Internasional*, officially published the very different scheme entitled Idiom Neutral. Idiom Neutral was reformed in 1907, and in 1908 the same body, under the name of *Academia pro Interlingua*, adopted Latino sine Flexione. The other great body engaged in work of a similar description, the "Delegation for the Adoption of an International Language," has remained faithful to its chosen language Ido. But Ido itself has not remained unmodified since its birth in 1907, and only in comparatively recent years has it begun to acquire the semblance of stability. The aim of the workers in these bodies is by careful comparison to select the language best suited for the purpose, and then to improve this language by introducing such changes as may seem advisable. The aim of the Esperantists is quite different: merely to use and extend the use of the language they already possess. Idists have recognized the distinct nature of these aims, and some of them have regarded the split between Esperanto and Ido as all to the good, through the division of labour that it has involved—Esperantists winning widespread adherence to the idea of international language, and Idists working towards linguistic perfection and "waiting for the time when the world will recognize the necessity for adopting the most efficient type of international language."[1]

3. Closely connected with these facts is a third distinction of importance, namely, the greater reliance on, and greater explicitness of, *principles* in the case of most recent languages, as compared with the relative empiricism of Esperanto. In the construction of the

---

[1] *E.g.* Dyer, *op. cit.*, p. 67 ; cf. Guérard, *op. cit.*, p. 189.

vocabulary of Esperanto, for instance, Zamenhof, though in the main guided by the idea of the greatest internationality, seems to have made no attempt at *strict* application of this or any other principle. He himself used the language (even to the extent of writing verse in it) for about six years before its publication, and during this time it *grew* under his hand, and some of these later growths—which were of course incorporated in the first text-books—are, as he himself expressly states,[1] of a kind that would probably never have occurred to him had he confined himself to theory. When Esperanto left Zamenhof's study to struggle for an existence in the outside world, it was already in a sense a living language, since it had been in prolonged daily use in the hands of its inventor.

A similar contrast between theoretic and empiric methods marks the history of the languages after their first publication. The contrast is well expressed by Dyer [2] in his comparison of Esperanto and Ido:

"The method of Esperanto is to leave the introduction of new words to the taste or necessity of the individual authors. If the arbitrary choice of the author meets with favour (is copied by other authors) the Lingva Komitato (the Esperanto language committee) may sooner or later officialize it. In Ido, the members of the Akedemio (the corresponding Idist institution) study each proposed new word in the light of the different forms of the word found in the various languages, together with the various definitions, and then introduce the word into the vocabulary. In other words, the method of Esperanto is to construct the vocabulary by individual use, that of Ido is scientifically controlled evolution."

[1] See Privat, *op. cit.*, p. 67.   [2] *Op. cit.*, p. 72.

These facts, like those indicated under (2), seem to be the inevitable consequences of the different mental attitudes of those concerned. Zamenhof and most of his followers are primarily interested in the use of their language for an ulterior purpose. The majority of those who have invented or concerned themselves with other schemes are primarily interested in the constructive manipulation or improvement of the language as an end in itself.

4. This difference of attitude involves another difference that has been of importance in the history of the languages concerned. Esperantists being either uninterested in purely linguistic questions or agreed that no definite changes in the language can be made, there is no room for serious internal disagreement as to the structure or growth of the language. We have already examined (p. 164) some of the psychological conditions of this fact, and have shown that they are probably connected to a considerable extent with Zamenhof's own attitude and character. Zamenhof himself submitted to the same restrictions as other Esperantists and abandoned all special power of control. The primarily linguistic interest underlying most other movements affords, on the contrary, ample opportunity for personal disputes as regards the adoption of this or that modification. Every individual has some justification for the assertion of his own views. The leaders of the various movements have, in particular—unlike Zamenhof—been very insistent on their own rights. The dissensions that brought about the fall of Volapük were chiefly due to a rebellion of the *Kadem bevünetik volupüka* and its leader Kerckhoffs against Schleyer's claims to absolute supremacy. In the subsequent history of the Academy, the changes

to which we referred in (2) were largely the result of
disputes between rival presidents, each fresh leader
asserting his own preferences as soon as he came to
power.[1] In the Delegation also there have been many
violent quarrels of a personal nature. Of Couturat,
for instance, Guérard writes: "For seven years he
flung excommunications broadcast, on conservatives
who refused to follow him, on progressives who went
one step ahead of him. . . . He had become that most
uncompromising of men: the infallible pope of a small
schismatic church."[2]

Owing to the exceptionally favourable father-regarding attitude caused by Zamenhof's renunciation of
power, together with the general agreement to accept
the language as it was and the concentration upon an
ulterior philanthropic aim, Esperantists were fortunately
able to avoid internal quarrels of this nature (though of
course they freely indulged their indignation against
the "traitor" de Beaufront and many of his fellow
Idists).

The Idist schism probably brought about the de-
fection of those who for one reason or another were
unable to renounce their own claims to power and
were incapable of looking upon Zamenhof as an ideal
beneficent father (de Beaufront himself as leader of
the movement in France gave many signs of restiveness
before he broke away).[3] It was the successful solution
of the Œdipus complex in the case of the majority of
Zamenhof's followers that enabled Esperantists successfully to weather a storm very similar to that which had
wrecked Volapük eighteen years before.

---

[1] Guérard, *op. cit.*, p. 141.   [2] *Ibid.*, p. 149.
[3] Cf. Privat, *op. cit.*, pp. 142 ff.

M

IV

THE ULTIMATE PSYCHOLOGICAL APPEAL OF INTERNATIONAL LANGUAGE

Hitherto we have been concerned with the description of some of the more striking features of the international language movement and with an attempt at a psychological exploration of these features in terms of mechanisms at the allo-erotic level.   In order to obtain a more complete psychological understanding of the phenomena, we must now proceed to an examination of certain more obscure factors connected with the more primitive Narcissistic and auto-erotic levels of the mind.   By anticipation we may state immediately that the castration complex and anal erotism will reveal themselves as among the most important of these factors.

In his paper on " The Madonna's Conception through the Ear," [1] Ernest Jones has indicated some important respects in which the function of speech is connected with the castration complex and with anal erotism. Speech, as he there shows, is for the unconscious mind in certain ways identical with life, creative power and God (the Logos doctrine), the tongue being a symbol of the phallus, while absence of speech (dumbness) is equivalent to impotence and death.   The function of speech, like that of breathing, blowing and the vocal production of sound in general, is also identified with the passing of flatus, while the reproductive and the anal elements combine together in the idea of gaseous fertilization, according to which impregnation takes place by the passing of flatus from father to mother.

---

[1] Chap. VIII of *Essays in Applied Psycho-Analysis.*

This idea of gaseous fertilization, he then proceeds to show, is in the nature of a reaction-formation to the idea of castration; it is the extreme antithesis to castration or impotence, inasmuch as it represents the very acme of (fertilizing) power.

Some additional facts pointing very strongly to the existence of an intimate connection between the ideas of speech and of phallic potency have also been brought forward by the present writer.[1]

In the light of all this evidence (to which the reader must be here referred) it would seem abundantly clear that linguistic power—whether of active speech or of understanding—is, in some of its aspects at least, unconsciously regarded as a representative or substitute for sexual power, and that linguistic inability stands in a similar relationship to sexual impotence or frigidity. Speaking in terms of conation we may say that linguistic activities are to some extent sublimations of sexual activities—a conclusion that accords well with Sperber's view concerning the sexual origin of speech [2] (a view which, we may note, is in essential harmony with that of so excellent a philologist as Jespersen).[3] In terms of affect—we may say again that the satisfaction derived from successful linguistic performance is to some extent a displacement of sexual satisfaction, while the pain of linguistic failure is a displacement of the pain of sexual impotence, and is able to draw upon the very strong conations associated with the castration complex.

If this view is correct, we must surely suppose that this equivalence of the linguistic with the sexual holds

[1] " A Note on the Phallic Significance of the Tongue and of Speech. *International Journal of Psycho-analysis*, 1925, VI, p. 209.

[2] " Uber den Einfluss sexueller Momente auf Entstehung und Entwicklung der Sprache," *Imago*, I, 1912, p. 405.

[3] *Language*, pp. 416 ff.

good, not only of speech in our native language, but also of our attempts to speak in foreign tongues. Indeed, so far as most adults are concerned, it is probably with regard to foreign languages that this equivalence produces its most marked effects, especially on the negative side. The use of our native tongue has become for most of us a humdrum everyday matter in which our abilities have become fairly accurately adjusted to our needs; a matter in which we customarily experience neither the joy of power nor the pain of incapacity. To experience the pleasure of success and the distress of failure in dealing with our mother tongue, we must belong to the relatively small class of those who attempt the more difficult linguistic feats, such as oratory or literary work, or those who suddenly endeavour to perform something more complex than that for which their previous training and habits have prepared them (as in the case of the more or less illiterate person who is suddenly called upon to write a letter). But when we attempt to speak or understand a foreign tongue, all this is changed; there is immediately a very marked increase in the affective value of all linguistic processes. Successful speech or understanding, from being nearly neutral in feeling, becomes distinctly pleasant (the more so, of course, the less we know the language), while failure to express our meaning seems to oppress us with a painful sense of impotence or inferiority.[1]

---

[1] There are, however, important individual and national differences in the reaction to this situation. In the German, for instance, the positive reactions are more marked than the negative. He is, broadly speaking, not seriously inhibited by the pains of failure ; his sense of inferiority is not so overwhelmingly stimulated by initial mistakes as to prevent him from persevering in his efforts, while, on the other hand, his sense of power and superiority seems greatly gratified by success. Compared with him, the

The more languages we know, the greater our sense of power derived from this unconscious source (and the greater of course our real capacity in many respects); the less we know of foreign languages, the greater our sense of inferiority arising from this same source, provided of course either that external circumstances are such as to make us realize our ignorance or that we are aware of falling below the cultural standard set us by our ego-ideal in this respect.

We are now in a position to appreciate one of the most important of the ways in which an international language appeals to the Unconscious. If the acquirement of each fresh language constitutes an additional gratifying manifestation of power (in the last resort

---

Englishman is as a rule a poor linguist because he is liable to be very greatly oppressed by a sense of inferiority whenever he fails.

The cause of such differences is probably complex in nature, but it is fairly clear that some factors of importance are connected with the social, historical and political implications of the language concerned. On the one hand, the Englishman's liability to inferiority feelings concerning foreign languages (which is perhaps only a particular manifestation of a very general tendency to linguistic inhibition) may possibly be due in part to the composite nature of his own language, and the fact that, as Ernest Jones has shown (*op. cit.*, p. 391 ff.) there tends to be a struggle between the Anglo-Saxon elements, which are endowed with greater emotional value, and the more delicate and aristocratic French elements, in favour of which the Anglo-Saxon elements have so often to be suppressed. Certainly the fact that French is the language of greater refinement and culture, plays to-day an important rôle in the fear which many English people have of using that language and of making mistakes in so doing.

On the other hand, native language, as we have seen, tends to be identified with the country in which it is spoken, so that patriotic sentiments may apply to one's native tongue as well as to one's native country, and the association of the English tongue with England is (for various political and historical reasons into which we need not enter) a closer one than that of the German language with Germany. Englishmen are, as a rule, prouder of their language than are Germans of theirs. Indeed, the Englishman tends to look down with a certain amount of arrogance upon the majority of foreign tongues; and this tendency provides him with a ready way of protecting himself against his feeling of inferiority. He can always fall back on the superiority

sexual power) and diminishes the sense of inferiority (based ultimately on the fear of sexual impotence or castration), it is clear that the knowledge of a universal language which would enable its possessor to understand and be understood by the inhabitants of all the world would afford access to the completest possible satisfaction on this plane, being inferior only to the manifestly impossible alternative of a knowledge of *all* living tongues.

Even to those already acquainted with a number of living languages, the use of a universal language appeals as a means of completing, and, so to speak, of rounding off their linguistic achievements. It is for this reason probably that international language often makes a strong appeal even to those who, in virtue of their

of English and England, and even persuade himself that to speak a foreign language is unpatriotic. The present writer remembers having been rebuked by a distinguished fellow-countryman for his efforts to talk a foreign language to a waiter, on the ground that "one shouldn't encourage the foreigners." This contrast in the attitude of English and Germans was well shown in the war, for the Germans seem to have persisted throughout in their study of English and French, whereas the English tended to look upon any interest in the German language as suspicious, and in extreme (though not so very infrequent) cases regarded it as " their duty to forget all the German they ever knew."

The Frenchman tends to react somewhat in the same manner as the Englishman, but carries the process a stage further. Secure in the possession of a language which—with fluctuations—has been the chief medium of European culture for several centuries, he feels that he is definitely absolved from the necessity of learning fóreign tongues. The exaggerated reaction of Englishmen in time of war is to quite a considerable extent a normal feature of the Frenchman's attitude, who feels that it would be degrading for him to struggle with the difficulties of a foreign tongue. Under the influence of this motive, a Frenchman will sometimes reveal an astonishing capacity to remain ignorant of another tongue which he may have heard about him for many years. His attitude towards his language is moreover paralleled by that towards his country, for having (as he would appear to think) been fortunate enough to be born in France, he is under no necessity to travel, and thus tends to avoid putting himself in a position to arouse feelings of inferiority in connection with his ignorance of foreign languages.

knowledge of other tongues, might appear to be least in need of it.   Thus, to mention two names only, the idea of a universal auxiliary tongue has aroused warm interest in so erudite a professional linguist and philologist as Jespersen and so gifted an amateur of languages as the late Sir William Ramsay—both men of quite exceptional polyglot knowledge and ability.   A personal friend of mine, who was until his death a prominent leader of the Esperanto movement, exhibited this tendency very strongly.   In his extensive travels he always made a point of acquiring as much knowledge as possible of the language of the country in which he found himself, and would have none of the excuses with which an ordinary tourist or linguist is apt to content himself for remaining ignorant of many of the minor languages; he would scorn for instance to talk Spanish in Catalonia or French in Brittany.[1]

There are two subsidiary, but nevertheless very important ways in which international language tends to increase our sense of power and lessen our feelings of inferiority.   In the first place, an international and artificial language, such as Esperanto or Ido, is very much easier to learn than are any languages that have acquired their present form through natural evolution.

[1] This condition being—of course to a minor degree—fairly common among the users of international language, there would seem to be at present very little ground for the fear expressed by opponents, that international language would diminish the interest in other tongues.   At present, only those who are interested in language—*i.e.* are in the last resort stimulated by unconscious motives such as we have here been considering—take up the study of Esperanto or Ido.   If, say, Esperanto were to become an obligatory subject in schools, the case might of course be different ; though even here we must reckon with the possibility that the study of Esperanto—admirably adapted as this would be to arouse an interest in the principles and structure of language in general—would lead to the formation or arousal of such unconscious motives in many people who would otherwise not have manifested them.

There is an absence of that bewildering wealth of grammatical and idiomatical variety which makes these latter languages so hard to acquire and so perilous to use by all who have not been familiar with them from their earliest years. At the same time, by a number of ingenious but simple devices, artificial language permits of great delicacy of expression with a minimum of knowledge and a minimum of intellectual effort. The fact that everything is permissible in Esperanto, so long as it is logical and is carried out in accordance with a few simple rules, makes it possible for every one to try experiments in the use and creation of linguistic forms; experiments that are quite impossible (except perhaps to a few specially endowed individuals) in the evolved languages, where convention carries far more weight than logic. All this gives a sense of freedom and of achieving much with little effort, that is very highly gratifying to those whose desire for power seeks a linguistic channel; it induces a psychic condition the very opposite of that sense of baffled impotence which besets the foreigner moving warily among the innumerable traps and pitfalls due to the illogicalities and inconsistencies of national language.

In the second place, an international artificial language places every one on the same footing. In the case of any natural language, those to whom this language is a mother-tongue have an undoubted advantage over those to whom it is an acquired idiom; an advantage which is apt to call forth feelings of superiority on the one part and feelings of inferiority on the other. The former feelings are indeed seldom openly manifested by cultured persons, being checked from motives of politeness or of sympathy, but free expression is sometimes given to them by such of the uneducated as seldom meet with foreigners. The feelings of inferiority are, however, felt in some degree by everyone who is compelled to speak in a foreign tongue (except in so far as they may be compensated in such ways as we have indicated).[1] The fear that at any moment it is possible to make some slip or break some linguistic convention, which may make one ridiculous in the eyes of one's interlocutor, is apt to cause serious inhibitions to very many persons—inhibitions which owe their potency largely to the fact that they have deep-lying unconscious roots.[2]

In the case of an artificial language this subjection of one of the speakers to an inevitable disadvantage is removed. Both the speakers have acquired the language; to neither is it a mother tongue, and even if mistakes are made, they appear less ridiculous and more forgivable to both parties; the painful feelings of inferiority are absent or are much reduced in intensity. The situation is similar in this respect to the case where two persons of different language are talking in a third natural language, which is the native tongue of neither of them—with the great additional advantage, however, that in the case of the artificial international language difficulties and mistakes are likely to be fewer, owing to the much greater ease with which such a language can be learnt. That the abolition or reduction of inferiority feeling due to this factor of both parties being on an equal footing is one of very real importance, will, I think, be admitted by all who have had an opportunity of comparing international gatherings in which only the natural tongues are spoken, with those in which the proceedings are in Esperanto.

[1] Page 180, note.   [2] Cf. below, page 201.

V

BABEL AND THE DIVERSITY OF TONGUES

We have by now, it may be hoped, made out a plausible case—to those acquainted with psychoanalysis—that international language owes some of its attractiveness to the fact that it gratifies in a highly sublimated form the desire for sexual potency, and serves as a reaction formation to the fear of impotence or castration. We have arrived at this conclusion by interpreting the observable phenomena concerning the international language movement in the light of psychological and ethnological evidence concerning language in general. We may, by way of concluding this portion of our argument, endeavour to strengthen our position by appeal to such scanty folkloristic evidence as seems to bear more directly upon our particular linguistic problem—the question of the diversity of natural tongues and the possibility of overcoming the mutual incomprehensibility of different sections of mankind that arises therefrom.

There exists one legend concerning the diversity of tongues which has been of outstanding importance for Western thought. I refer of course to the Biblical story of the Tower of Babel.[1] Workers in the cause of international language have not unnaturally regarded themselves—in seriousness or in fancy—as engaged in the task of undoing the mischief that was wrought on that inauspicious occasion when Jehovah confounded the languages of those engaged in the building of the Tower. Thus one of the most popular books advocating Esperanto in the English language, is entitled *The*

---

[1] Genesis xi, 1–9.

Passing of Babel; while on the other hand objections are still sometimes advanced against any international language on the ground of its impiety, as contrary to the will of God as manifested at Babel. That the legend makes a very powerful general appeal is shown by the great wealth of detail with which it became adorned in later Jewish tradition and the readiness with which it seems to have been incorporated into the mythology of very different peoples (for the similarity between a good many of the relevant legends in several different parts of the world is in this case too great to allow us to suppose that Christian or Jewish influences have not been at work).

Now Lorenz in his study of the Titan Motive in Mythology,[1] has shown that this legend belongs to a class of story concerned with the storming of heaven, a theme which represents a cosmical projection of the father hatred connected with the Œdipus complex, and of which the well-known history of Otos and Ephialtes, who endeavoured to reach heaven by piling Ossa on Olympus and Pelion on Ossa, represents the analogue in classical mythology. The hostile intention of the tower builders is well brought out in the later Jewish traditions to which we have referred. For from these we learn "that the enterprise of the tower was flat rebellion against God, though the rebels were not at one in their aims. Some wished to scale heaven and there wage war with the Almighty in person or set up their idols to be worshipped in His stead; others limited their ambition to the more modest scheme of damaging the celestial vault by showers of spears and arrows. Many, many years was the tower in building. It reached

[1] " Das Titanenmotiv in der Allgemeinen Mythologie," *Imago,* II, 1913, pp. 48 ff.

so high that at last a bricklayer took a whole year to ascend to the top. . . . Day and night the work never slackened; and from their dizzy height they shot heavenwards arrows, which returned to them dabbled with blood; so they cried 'We have slain all who are in heaven.'"[1] The high tower motive, which is here so vividly portrayed, is at the same time a symbolic expression of the process of erection, similar to that found in Jacob's dream of the ladder reaching from earth to heaven,[2] in the very common dreams of flying and climbing, and in the not infrequent stories of the Jack and the Beanstalk type, though in many of these latter instances (including Jacob's dream) the act of coitus is also symbolized through the rhythmical movements of climbing.

The successful storming of heaven thus represents defiance of the father and gratification of the sexual desires. Failure of the enterprise, as in the Babel story, represents the revenge of the threatened father. Psychoanalysis has prepared us for the form that this revenge will take; we know well that in the unconscious mind the punishment appropriate to father defiance is castration. Now it would seem probable that in the Biblical story and its later elaborations the castration finds a fourfold symbolization. The first and most obvious symbol is the destruction of the tower itself. In connection with this we may note with Lorenz[3] that later versions point to a tradition that Jehovah destroyed the tower by means of a strong wind. Ernest Jones[4] reminds us that here we have another allusion to the flatus—breath—castration—sexual-power associa-

---

[1] Frazer : *Folklore in the Old Testament*, Vol. I, p. 364.
[2] Rank, *Das Inzestmotiv in Dichtung und Sage*, p. 302.
[3] *Op. cit.*, pp. 51, 52.   [4] *Op. cit.*, p. 354.

tions to which his paper is devoted, the myth of Bable being in this respect, as Lorenz had already pointed out, allied to the destruction of the walls of Jericho by the blowing of trumpets. We may note also that, according to Hyginus, it is Hermes, the god of the winds, who is responsible for *discord* and *diversity of speech* among mankind,[1] and that in the Polynesian version of the Titan story the wind god Tawhiri-ma-tea assists his parents in the Titanic struggle and *scatters* far and wide his brothers by means of the tempest that he raises.[2] In these three features, *scattering*, *discord* and *diversity of speech*, we have the three other symbols of castration that are operative in the Babel story. All three have obviously much in common; they are all forms of separation and all are probably variations on the theme of dismemberment.[3] In the first case there is dismemberment of the group by separation in space, in the second case there is dismemberment through the mutual hostility of the members,[4] in the third case dismemberment through mutual incomprehensibility. They differ from ordinary symbols of castration in that the castration complex as expressed therein, instead of referring merely to the individual, is projected on to the whole of humanity. They thus bear much the

---

[1] See Frazer, *op. cit.*, p.384.

[2] Lorenz, *ibid.*, p. 52.

[3] *Op. cit. International Journal of Psycho-Analysis*, 1925, VI, p. 211.

[4] This hostility corresponds, of course, on the Darwin-Atkinson-Freud hypothesis, to the struggle between the brothers who have slain (or would have slain) the primal father. It also represents a projection of the internal struggle in the minds of the rebellious sons—a struggle between hate of the father and revolt against him on the one hand, and love of him, fear of him and obedience to him on the other ; a projection which, as Lorenz has shown, finds very full expression in the Titan myths, as a struggle between two groups of Titans, one of which fights against the gods and the other on the side of the gods.

same relation to the usual symbolical expressions of the castration idea, as the flood legends bear to the symbols of individual birth.[1] That there should be such a displacement from the individual body to the "body" (note the word) of mankind at large is not surprising when we bear in mind the extremely frequent use of the analogy between the individual and the social organism, by thinkers both of the past and of the present.

It is probably no mere coincidence that the comparison between the dismemberment of the state through civil strife and the dismemberment (castration) of an individual finds vivid portrayal in *Titus Andronicus*, that play which, as we have elsewhere indicated,[2] is so intimately concerned with the castration complex in other respects. The passage concerned also contains the ideas of scattering by wind, noise ("uproar") and difficulties of speech or of adequately conveying one's meaning, as well as a direct reference to castration (Sinon, who mutilated himself as part of the stratagem to enter Troy).

MARCUS: You sad-faced men, people and sons of Rome,
   By uproar severed, like a flight of fowl
    Scattered by wind and high tempestuous gusts,
   O! let me teach you how to knit again
    This scattered corn into one mutual sheaf,
   These broken limbs again into one body;
   Lest Rome herself be bane unto herself,
   And she whom mighty kingdoms curtsey to,
    Like a forlorn and desperate *castaway*
   Do shameful execution on herself.
   But if my frosty signs and chaps of age,
   Grave witnesses of true experience,
    Cannot induce you to attend my words,

[1] See Rank, *Psychoanalytische Beiträge zur Mythenforschung*, pp. 147 ff.
[2] *International Journal of Psycho-analysis*, 1925, VI, p. 209.

(*To* LUCIUS.)

> *Speak*, Rome's dear friend, as erst our ancestor,
>   When with his solemn *tongue* he did *discourse*
> To lovesick Dido's sad attending ear
>   The story of that baleful burning night
> When subtle Greeks surprised King Priam's Troy;
>   Tell us what *Sinon* hath *bewitched our ears*,
> Or who hath brought the fatal engine in
>   That gives our Troy, our Rome, this *civil wound*.
> My heart is not compact of flint or steel,
> But floods of tears will *drown my oratory*
> *And break my very utterance.*

ACT V, sc. 3.

The introduction here of Sinon is itself of some interest, for it points to incest with the mother as the cause of castration. Sinon's story was that the Greeks had constructed the wooden horse as an atonement for the stealing of the Palladium, the image of the goddess which guaranteed the inviolability of Troy (*i.e.* as an atonement for mother incest), and he persuaded the Trojans that if they drew the horse into the city, this inviolability would be restored. In reality it is pretty clear that Sinon's mutilation is the genuine atonement; the horse, on the other hand, plays the part of the phallus which again commits the crime of mother incest in conveying the armed men into the city, for the taking and sacking of a city is a symbol of rape—ultimately of the mother.[1] As if to make clear this latter point, Electra, the mother of Dardanus, the founder of Troy, on learning of the city's destruction, tore out her hair in grief and was placed among the stars.

The dependence upon the Œdipus complex of the castration symbolized by the diversity of tongues is

---

[1] Cp. Rank, " Um Städte werben," *Zeitschrift f. Psychoanalyse*, 1914 II, p. 50.

indicated pretty clearly also by certain stories of the origin of differences of language which would appear to be quite independent of Greek or Biblical tradition.[1] Thus among the Kachcha Nagas, a hill tribe of Assam, there is a story of a lost princess and a python, very reminiscent of the European stories in which the father is symbolized as a dragon who is about to slay the princess (mother). A princess who is the daughter of the king of men disappears, and a prolonged search is made for her by all the king's subjects. At length they discover an enormous python and proceed to attack it with spear and sword, but even as they strike their dialect is changed.

The Kukis, another tribe of Assam, think that the diversity of tongues first arose in the case of three boys who were engaged in hunting a rat, although their grandfather had forbidden them to do so.

The Maidu Indians of California have a story that diversity of language arose when they were preparing to have a "burning," which, as Frazer says, probably means "a performance of the shamans who danced to the light of a fire kindled by the friction of wood and who professed to walk through this fire unscathed." This playing with fire is, as we know, a sexual symbol, and is often intimately connected with the rebellion of the son against the father, as the myth of Prometheus testifies.[2]

The Encounter Bay tribe of South Australia trace both the origin and the diversity of language to an ill-tempered old woman named Wurruri, who used to walk about with a big stick ("woman with the penis") and scatter the fire around when other people were

---

[1] See Frazer, *op. cit.*, pp. 384 ff.
[2] Cf. Abraham, *Traum und Mythus*, pp. 26 ff.

sleeping (note the recurrence of the fire theme). When she died, everyone was so pleased that a feast was held and everybody regaled themselves on her flesh, and having done so began to speak intelligibly for the first time. But men spoke different languages according to the part of her body that they happened to consume.

Cannibalism in this connection reminds us of *Titus Andronicus*, the story of Tereus, the eating of the serpents' tongues to understand the language of animals, etc.[1] No doubt the frequency of the theme is due to the fact that both eating (of parents by children and children by parents) and castration are often recurring features of the Œdipus complex (sometimes too it is just the penis that is eaten, as in the case of Osiris). But it may well be that the connection ultimately depends upon deep-lying mechanisms of the oral stage which have not as yet been fully explored.

VI

PENTECOST AND THE GIFT OF TONGUES

If the story of Babel has become the accepted account of the origin of the diversity of tongues, the Pentecostal gift of tongues [2] has often been held to constitute in some sense a providential antithesis to the divine punishment involved in the earlier incident. As Grotius has put it: "Poena linguarum dispersit homines; donum linguarum dispersos in unum populum collegit." This is an attitude that has been adopted by a good many advocates of international

---

[1] See *International Journal of Psycho-analysis ; loc. cit.*
[2] Described in Acts ii, 1-13.

N

language, the function of which has been likened to a modern "gift of tongues."

Biblical scholars are now, it would seem, pretty well agreed that Luke's description in Acts rests upon a misunderstanding (it was probably written some sixty years after the event), and that what really happened was a speaking of unintelligible jargon, rather than of foreign languages—in technical terms glossolalia, not xenoglossia. This would bring the occurence into line with the other cases of tongue speech referred to in Acts and in Corinthians, which were undoubtedly of the former variety, and also renders more comprehensible the remark of some of the bystanders to the effect that the Apostles were drunk. Glossolalia was, and still is, a recognized feature of certain religious manifestations, and has been studied psycho-analytically by Pfister.[1] From the purely psychological point of view there is perhaps no very great difference between the two kinds of speech; glossolalia is probably only a form of would-be xenoglossia, for Pfister found,[2] as one of the more general motives underlying the phenomenon, the desire to understand some (foreign) language, from which many of the words were taken and distorted. This obviously links on to the motive of (linguistic) power that we have already studied. That we are moreover, here as before, ultimately concerned with sexual power, together with the ideas of breath and flatus connected therewith, has already been made clear by Ernest Jones in his paper on the Holy Ghost,[3] where it has been shown that the Holy Ghost in one of

[1] " Die Psychologische Enträtselung der religiösen Glossolalie und der automatischen Kryptographie," *Jahrbuch für psychoanalytische und psychopathologische Forschungen*, 1912, III, pp. 472, 730.
[2] *Ibid.*, p. 780.　　　　[3] *Op. cit.* p. 415.

its aspects represents the creative essence of the Father, the same power that manifested itself in the conception of the Madonna through the ear. Indeed, the "mighty rushing wind" and the "cloven tongues as of fire" would naturally lead us to expect that we are here concerned with essentially the same forces as those which we have hitherto encountered; only that in the present case the divine power is beneficent and not malignant, creative and not destructive. In the Pentecostal gift of tongues God of his own pleasure endows men with some of his own creative power, the gift of potency as symbolized in foreign speech; whereas at Babel, God used his power for the destruction of man's potency as symbolized in the same way—a typical contrast between the points of view of the Old and the New Testaments respectively. In the latter we have reached a stage of moral evolution at which the agelong conflict between Father and Son has, superficially at any rate, been brought to rest. The war of the gods and Titans has been terminated, not (as at an earlier stage) by the defeat and brutal subjection of the latter, but by a reconciliation between the combatants. At this later level of religious thought Prometheus is no longer castrated for stealing fire from heaven. There is no need to steal, for the divine fire is freely given by the Father to his children.

The attitude of those who have contrasted the destruction of Babel and the Gift of Tongues is therefore justified. The latter really constitutes a making good of the injury committed by the former. Sexual potency, in its displaced form as linguistic power, is abolished at Babel and re-created by means of the Pentecostal gift. In this gift the ability to speak to and to under-stand men of diverse speech is clearly an abolition of the curse of impotence, a creation of fresh sexual power. International language as a practical realization on a vast scale of this linguistic dream is admirably adapted to serve in modern life as a displacement of the same kind as that recorded by the writer of the Acts.

VII

THE CREATION AND USE OF INTERNATIONAL LANGUAGE

In dealing thus far with factors of the genital level, and particularly with the castration complex, we have throughout been implicitly aware of the existence of anal factors underlying the genital ones, but—relying on the fact that Ernest Jones has studied at length the connection between the anal and the genital elements here concerned—we have not examined closely the nature and function of these underlying anal factors. Now, however, it behoves us to point to one or two special ways in which anal factors seem to play a rôle of some importance in the international language movement. At the same time we shall have the opportunity of dealing with a few influences emanating from the genital or allo-erotic levels with which we have not yet dealt, or at which we have, at best, only cast a very rapid glance in passing.

If we accept Ernest Jones' conclusions, we must assume that there are anal factors underlying many of the ideas of potency with which we have been dealing. This is quite in accord with much that we have already learnt from psycho-analysis, which has taught us that (in the unconscious mind) genital potency is, in certain of its aspects, identified with potency of the excretory processes. The child takes pride in its excretory functions long before it is acquainted with the genital functions, and in the course of development these latter are, through displacement, invested with some of the affect originally attaching to the former. Thus the pride in the ability to create a child is to some extent derived from the early (and subsequently repressed) pride in the production of fæces, while the linguistic displacements that we have been considering represent substitute gratifications at both levels.

In view of the connection between speech, impregnation and flatus to which Ernest Jones has drawn attention, we can scarcely doubt that displaced anal affects (ultimately derived from the satisfaction gained by the production of fæces or flatus) play a part in the joy of *creating* an artificial language.

When we consider the really formidable nature of the task, and the fact that the creation of a language requires a linguistic knowledge and capacity possessed by very few, it is surprising to learn of the vast number of systems of international language that have at one time or another been prepared.[1] But it is perhaps a little less astonishing if we remember the very common nature of the underlying complexes and if we bear in mind also the psycho-analytic discovery that one of the features of certain well-marked types of anal character is dogged perseverance in the face of obstacles.[2]

The anal displacements involved in the impulse to create probably find expression not only in the creation of a language as a whole, but in the creation of new words, idioms or modes of expression—a form of linguistic activity for which, as we have seen above

---

[1] See Couturat and Leau, *Histoire de la Langue Universelle*, and the abbreviated account in Clark, *International Language*, p. 78.

[2] See Ernest Jones, *Papers on Psycho-Analysis*, 2nd ed., p. 667.

(p. 184), the use of an artificial language offers exceptional facilities; while, in the absence of a suitable linguistic medium or a sufficient linguistic knowledge, the same impulse under other circumstances probably plays a by no means unimportant part in glossolalia.

Infantile anal satisfaction is connected not only with the creation of fæces but also with the tendency to play with or manipulate the fæces. In all probability this manifestation of anal erotism also finds expression in the last-mentioned activities, which to some extent may be regarded as a kind of playing with language. In a few individuals (some of whom have been important in the history of international language) this tendency has found a more ambitious outlet in playing with the essential structure of the language itself (as opposed to the mere manipulation of linguistic forms according to existing rules), and thus has contributed largely to the desire to modify and reform the language, a desire which we have already studied rather fully from the point of view of the Œdipus complex. In virtue of the fact that these anal activities—both productive and manipulative—very early in life become connected with defiance (because they frequently lead to manifestations of disapproval on the part of parents or nurses), they very easily associate themselves with any tendencies to rebellion against authority that may be aroused at higher mental levels. In the present case, an association of this kind leads to reinforcement by these primitive impulses of the attitude towards the language that springs from displacements of the Œdipus complex. The modifying of the international language thus affords satisfaction in a displaced form at two levels:—at the level of the Œdipus complex, it signifies, as we have seen, defiance of the father (the creator of the language who forbids others to tamper with it) and incest with the mother (taking forbidden liberties with the language); on the anal-erotic level, it signifies the defiance of the nursery authorities by indulgence in the tabooed anal activities (linguistic creation or manipulation in unpermitted ways).[1]

If these positive manifestations of anal-erotism have played a significant part in the international language movement, so also have the forces that are concerned in the *repression* of anal-erotism. With regard to the last-mentioned example, for instance, just as, on the positive side, the desire to create or play with fæces reinforces the incest tendencies in their sublimated expression as a tendency to modify the language, so also, on the negative side, the inhibitions attaching to the anal manifestations add their strength to the inhibitions arising from the Œdipus complex; the inhibitions from the two sources work together in the maintenance of the attitude that the *Fundamento* is *netuŝebla*. It is forbidden (literally) to touch fæces or (metaphorically) to touch the mother, and the language is a symbol for both these objects.

Perhaps the most important effects of the anal

---

[1] The tendency to the creation of artificial languages by children or adolescents (such languages as have been studied by Jespersen, *op. cit.*, pp. 180 ff.) is undoubtedly connected with the defiance of authority, particularly with the desire for secrecy with regard to sexual subjects (cp. Tausk, " A Contribution to the Psychology of Child Sexuality," *International Journal of Psycho-Analysis*, 1924, V, p. 350). In virtue of this secrecy—the secret language even if overheard is unintelligible to the authorities—children reverse the position of inferiority in which they found themselves in infancy, when they did not yet fully understand the conversation of adults, or in which they may still find themselves when, as happens not infrequently in educated families, the parents resort to a foreign language in order not to be understood by their children. In addition to this, the use of the secret language affords of course, many satisfactions—genital and anal in level—to which we have already referred in dealing with international language.

repressions are to be found, however, not so much within the movement, as in the attitude of the outside public towards international language. It is a strange but indisputable fact that to a large number of cultured people the idea of an artificial language, especially when first encountered, is apt to appear distinctly repellent or *disgusting*. It is as a rule difficult to ascertain the true grounds of this disgust—any reasons that may be advanced by those who feel this emotion being for the most part quite palpably in the nature of rationalizations. It is pretty certain then that the emotion is aroused from some unconscious sources, and it would seem that the considerations we have just been making with regard to the co-operation of repressions affecting anal-erotism on the one hand and incest tendencies on the other may be able to throw light on the nature of these sources. If the creation of language is, as we have seen, unconsciously regarded as equivalent to the production of fæces or flatus, and if the manipulation of existing natural languages (such as is inevitably involved in the construction of an *a posteriori* artificial language) is similarly regarded as equivalent to playing with fæces, the arousal of disgust is no longer incomprehensible. It becomes still more intelligible when we add to the powerful repressions here involved the influence of the co-operative factors on the allo-erotic level. People who feel disgust at the idea of an artificial language will often discourse at length upon the "beauty" and "sanctity" of "natural languages," and regard with horror the idea of tampering with this sanctity in order to create an easy artificial language.[1]

[1] This insistence upon beauty is probably to some extent a reaction formation against the anal-erotic tendencies (cf. Jones, *op. cit.*, p. 678); a reaction formation which may be here placed in the service of the sublimation of the incest tendencies.

This process of tampering—in addition to its coprophilic significance—is, we may surmise, for many such persons the equivalent of an attack upon the mother, an attack all the more revolting because it is associated with the forbidden coprophilic tendencies and therefore probably conceived in terms of infantile sexual theories of the anal level, thus constituting what might quite appropriately be called a "pollution" of the mother.

Reactions of this kind are much more frequent in the case of persons of higher than of lower culture; indeed, such reactions probably constitute one of the chief causes of the fact that, as we noted before (p. 167), the international language movement has enjoyed comparatively little support from the more aristocratic and educated classes. The reason for the much greater frequency of this attitude of disgust among the latter class is, we may suggest, probably connected with the greater preoccupation of this class with linguistic matters. This greater preoccupation affords an opportunity for the displacement of the lower level tendencies into a linguistic field, in a way that is not so easy in the case of those whose activities are such as to give rise to fewer and less intense interests in linguistic questions; with these latter persons the corresponding displacements and reaction, formations must probably be sought outside the sphere of language.[1]

---

[1] We may note in passing that there is probably much truth in the views of those who attribute to linguistic factors considerable importance in the production of class hatred and class misunderstanding. The cultured are apt to feel toward the language and behaviour of the less educated a sort of disgust which is probably derived from anal sources. This is indicated very strikingly in a well-known passage from *Julius Cæsar* (Act I, sc. 2), which contains abundant allusions of a kind that has become familiar to us in this study. " The rabblement shouted and clapped their chopped hands, threw up their sweaty night-caps, and uttered such a deal of stinking breath because Cæsar

VIII

THE OBJECTIONS TO INTERNATIONAL LANGUAGE

This repulsion felt towards artificial language in the case of numerous cultured persons is often reinforced by certain additional factors, of which we may here refer to three, as being perhaps especially frequent and important. In the first place, the major natural languages, with their imposing literatures and traditions extending over many years, are eminently calculated to attract displacement of the tenderness, admiration and respect originally attaching to the mother. Regarded thus as the equivalents of the more idealised aspect of the mother, they contrast very markedly with artificial languages which possess but little literature and no traditions.[1]

In the second place language is, as we have more than once had occasion to remind the reader, very intimately connected with the country in which the language is spoken. This is especially true of an individual's own language, which therefore tends to attract to itself all the strong parent-regarding feelings which underlie the affection for one's native land. To use or to advocate an international language may thus

refused the crown, that it almost choked Cæsar, for he swooned and fell down at it ; and for mine own part, I durst not laugh, for fear of opening my lips and receiving the bad air."

The proletariat on their side are apt to regard the language of the cultured as finicky, emasculated and pedantic, and their persistence in linguistic usages that are deprecated at school or by their social superiors is probably due in part to a displacement of infantile tendencies to anal defiance.

[1] Thus an English objector once remarked—very appositely from this point of view—that to use Esperanto when one could use English would be " to forsake one's birthright for a mess of pottage." Note the implications of the words *birthright* and *mess*.

appear to indicate a lack of patriotic feeling, especially in the case of persons whose own languages (*e.g.* English or French) are already largely used for international purposes.

The third factor is Narcissistic in nature, and perhaps deserves a somewhat fuller treatment. A knowledge of foreign languages is nowadays generally demanded of educated persons and is itself regarded as a sign of culture, while the lack of such a knowledge is apt to reflect to some extent upon a person's cultural status and to give rise to corresponding feelings of inferiority in the person himself.[1]

The demand for an easy international auxiliary language is apt to produce an unpleasant realization of one's inevitable deficiences in this respect; it tends to make us recognize that at best we are only acquainted with a very few foreign languages out of the great number that exist, and that our knowledge even of those with which we have some acquaintance is often very deficient; that in fact the problem of learning foreign languages has definitely proved too difficult for us. The help offered by international language is therefore indignantly refused, for much the same reason that an elderly man will sometimes be angry if we offer to help him in putting on his coat. In both cases, the proffered assistance constitutes a painful reminder of infirmities.

That such a factor is really at work in the case of international language is indicated by a not infrequent experience of the present writer. On advocating Esperanto, he is met with the rather hurried, irritated and embarrassed reply: "I would much rather devote

---

[1] Both these feelings and the correlated feelings of superiority being of course ultimately connected with the ideas of potency considered in previous sections.

my time to the study of some national language," and the very obvious retort to the effect that the time required to gain a good working knowledge of Esperanto would suffice to give only the merest smattering of any national language then elicits sudden collapse, angry protestations or a rapid change of front of such a kind as to indicate that a sore spot had been touched, that the difficulty of acquiring foreign languages was a painful subject to the person in question and that his imperfect knowledge in this direction was a source of considerable uneasiness and even shame. This factor is of much less weight with persons of fewer cultural pretensions. For them it is no disgrace to be ignorant of foreign languages, and they can freely avail themselves of the benefits of Esperanto (with the delightful, and to them unaccustomed, sense of power that this gives), without the arousal of the feelings of inferiority to which—owing to a kind of intellectual snobbery—the more cultured are liable to be exposed.[1]

This relative immunity that in many countries distinguishes the less-cultured classes is perhaps shown to some extent by Frenchmen of all grades. Owing to the Frenchman's tendency to adopt a peculiar attitude of superiority towards foreign tongues—an attitude we have already noted in another connection—he is apt to feel the disgrace of linguistic ignorance

[1] Perhaps the most extreme form of intellectual snobbery of this kind manifests itself in the proposal to make Latin the official international language. The study of Latin is and has been for many centuries the privilege of the aristocratic and learned classes, and its adoption for international purposes to-day would necessarily be confined to the relatively few individuals who had sufficient time, opportunity and ability to master its difficulties. Latin has in the past really served the purpose of an international language among the cultured persons throughout Europe, and it is very natural that many scholars, mindful of this fact, should contemplate with distaste the substitution of an easy and democratic language such as Esperanto.

a good deal less keenly than are cultured persons of most other Western nations. It is very probably owing to this fact that the international language movement has in France, it would seem, gained the support of a larger proportion of cultured and aristocratic persons than in most other countries.

The anal repressions dealt with in the last section, together with the co-operating tendencies at higher levels that we have here considered, constitute formidable psychological obstacles to the widespread adoption of an international language. At the same time, however, they also operate in certain ways that are of assistance to the movement, and will perhaps do so still more in the future. On an earlier page we drew attention to the feelings of inferiority aroused by the fact that in speaking foreign languages we are liable at any moment to break some rule of grammar or syntax or some idiomatic convention, thus rendering ourselves ridiculous to the ears of natives. The embarrassment which the commission of such a slip may cause to many sensitive persons is probably due in the last resort to anal associations. In a case studied by myself, analysis revealed very clearly that the process of making slips of the tongue—"accidents" as the patient called them —was unconsciously equated to infantile "accidents" connected with the excretory processes.[1] I am inclined to believe that a similar identification applies in many instances to slips made in the case of foreign languages. It is now pretty generally recognized by psycho-analysts that anal factors often play a part in our attitude towards linguistic correctness, extending (to quote Ernest Jones[2])

---

[1] The actual nature of any particular slip would of course reveal some specific tendency as well.

[2] *Op. cit.*, p. 687.

"into the finest details of syntax and grammar."[1] This being the case, it would be surprising if these factors did not also play a part in our attitude towards foreign languages.

The commission of mistakes arouses disagreeable feelings owing to anal repression, not only in the person who is guilty of them, but also in the listener who is condemned to hear his native tongue (or some other language that he loves and admires) "murdered" by the clumsiness of some incompetent linguist. The scholarly schoolmaster who is "disgusted" by the "howlers" of the feebler Latinists among his pupils affords one striking example of this kind, but other cases are not hard to find. Indeed, it would seem that

---

[1] There seem to be few, if any, aspects of language into which the anal influences do not penetrate. Persons whose repression of anal-erotism takes on a linguistic form may be equally distressed by faulty accent or stress (false quantities), slipshod or incorrect pronunciation, mistakes of grammar or syntax (split infinitives), bad style, ugly or illegible handwriting and un-orthodox spelling. The connection between anal-erotism and spelling has not—so far as I am aware—been noted yet in psycho-analytic literature, but it has been observed by Cyril Burt in the course of his psychological studies on school children (*Mental and Scholastic Tests*, p. 293). I have myself recently enjoyed the opportunity of studying two cases presenting different types of anal character whose reactions to spelling and other linguistic matters afforded an exceptionally vivid contrast. *A* was of the retentive anal type, exceedingly careful as regards the spending of money, scrupulous as regards matters of cleanliness, regular in habits and disliking any change of routine, accustomed to spend a long time in the w.c. reading a newspaper ; he was very upset by any departure from linguistic convention, mistakes in spelling and grammar appearing to him to have betrayed a shocking lack of breeding. *B* was of the opposite " productive " type. Very generous and inclined to be extravagant, cleanly, but disliking routine even in matters of the toilet, spending the shortest possible time in the w.c. and never reading there, he wrote rapidly and fluently and with a certain disregard for syntax. He was extremely intolerant of orthographic conventions and would some-times spell a word in several different ways in the course of a single letter. The attitude underlying his bad spelling was undoubtedly due to a displace-ment of anal defiance, the continuance in a different field of a refusal to submit to " arbitrary " nursery restrictions with reference to the process of excretion.

a widespread tendency to an attitude of this kind would constitute a very serious obstacle to the adoption of Latin or of any living national language as an international auxiliary tongue. The same applies also in a large measure to any possible simplifications of such languages as might be adopted for international use—such as Ogden's recent proposal for "Basic English." Students of the international language problem are for the most part in agreement that simplifications of existing languages (such as those that have been actually proposed in the case of Latin or English[1]) would be regarded by very many as in the nature of a mutilation or desecration of the languages concerned and would therefore be liable to meet with great opposition from the more educated classes. This opposition would indeed quite possibly be even greater than that which, as we have just seen, is encountered by a frankly artificial language.

From these last-mentioned points of view, there may accrue a certain advantage to the international language movement. Owing to its comparative ease, a speaker may more easily avoid the mistakes which cause embarrassment owing to the coprophilic associations; and owing to its neutrality, even if mistakes are made, these are less likely to appear to the listener as in the nature of an attack or pollution than would be the case with a national tongue.

[1] Shakespeare's phrase, " abusing of the King's English," points, however, to resistances—of the kind we have already considered—rising primarily from the Œdipus level. Nevertheless, on this level, it may be possible to look upon the proposed international use of English—even in a simplified form—as an extension of the power and glory of the parents, much as in the case of the enlargement of the British Empire ; and satisfaction on this score may, of course, in some cases outweigh the objections on the anal level.

IX

FORMS OF INTERNATIONAL LANGUAGE

Finally we may note very briefly certain ways in which anal factors have played a part in the actual process of construction of the various artificial languages that have been proposed. In the history of these languages it is possible to discern the influence of various conflicting tendencies. Thus a desire for wealth and variety of forms has competed with the desire for brevity and conciseness, the desire for linguistic purity with the desire for the maximum of neutrality and internationality, and the desire for logical consistency with the desire for ease of comprehension at first sight. It would seem from what we know of the linguistic manifestations of anal-erotism that coprophilic traits may have exerted a not inconsiderable influence upon the choice of any given author in favour of one or the other of these alternatives.

Thus, the more positive aspects of coprophilia would lead to a desire to create a language very rich in vocabulary and in grammar. Hence, in all probability, arose, for instance, the extraordinary project of the earliest British worker in the field, Sir Thomas Urquhart, a project which must be seen to be believed.[1] This project appeared in 1653 under the resounding title of :—

" Logopandekteision

or, an Introduction to the Universal Language, digested into these Six Several Books:

Neaudethaumata	Chryseomystes
Chrestasebeia	Neleodicastes
Cleronomaporia	Philoponauxesis,"

[1] And which certainly deserves to be studied in the abstract given by Clark (*op. cit.*, pp. 87 ff.) by all who are interested in the subject.

and was, we are told, "given out to two separate printers, one alone not being fully able to hold his quill a-going." In it the author expounds in detail the superiority of his new language over all others. This superiority, it would appear, rests chiefly upon the fact that for each department of speech it has a greater variety of forms; thus it has eleven cases, four numbers (singular, dual, plural and redual), eleven genders ("wherein likewise it exceedeth all other languages") and seven moods, while "verbs, mongrels, participles and hybrids have all of them ten tenses, besides the present, which number no language else is able to attain to." The language was also very rich on the emotional side, for "as its interjections are more numerous, so they are more emphatical in their respective expressions of passions than that part of speech is in any other language whatsoever," while "of all languages [it] is the most compendious in compliment, and consequently fittest for Courtiers and Ladies."

As a contrast to this joy in linguistic exuberance we may compare " Pan Roman " (later called " Universal "), the scheme of Dr. Molenaar, published in 1903. Dr. Molenaar is very proud of the "spareness" of his language, which aims throughout at the greatest possible brevity, particularly perhaps in its use of vowel sounds. To many others, however, we are told by Guérard,[1] the language has a "close-cropped air, which caused it to be compared to a musician just out of jail, or, more poetically, to a cathedral after an iconoclastic riot" (note the castration symbolism). In a similar way, Guérard tells us[2] that Professor Peano, the author of "Latino sine Flexione," "carried the principle of grammatical economy to the extreme of niggardliness."

[1] *Op. cit.*, p. 143.　　　　[2] *Op. cit.*, p. 163.

O

In general the tendency during the recent history of international language has undoubtedly been in the direction of "spareness" rather than exuberance. Thus Esperanto is much simpler than Volapük, and Ido is perhaps in some respects simpler than Esperanto. Zamenhof's original plans for Esperanto were much more complex than those that he eventually adopted on publication of the language. But this increasing linguistic asceticism is perhaps not achieved without a real effort of renunciation, and at least one former Esperantist, Kürschner, published in 1900 a language which was a good deal more complicated than Esperanto, possessing, for instance, several conjugations of the verb.[1]

Dr. Molenaar's attitude serves to reveal not only the struggle between conciseness and expansiveness, but also that between purity and neutrality. To him, "a mixed language like Esperanto is a hotch-potch, hideous and barbaric."[2] As the name of his own language indicates, he will have none but roots of purest Latin origin, and in this he has of course been followed by many other inventors.[3] The demand for purity and the abhorrence of linguistic admixtures (contrast Urquhart's "mongrels" and "hybrids") together, in Molenaar's case, with insistence on the utmost parsimony, leave little doubt as to the reaction-formations to anal-erotism that are here involved.[4]

---

[1] Clark, *op. cit.*, p. 86.

[2] Guérard, *op. cit.*, p. 144.

[3] Americans are wont to allow themselves much greater linguistic freedom than do English. They show little or no dislike, for instance, to the combination in neologisms of Latin and Greek roots, a practice to which most cultured Englishmen object. Perhaps the very general linguistic inhibitions which characterize the English may be to some extent dependent on a reaction-formation to anal-erotic tendencies.

[4] Cp. Jones, *op. cit.*, p. 686.

The third of the above-mentioned conflicts—that between logical consistency and immediate ease of understanding[1] —is one in which it is probable that anal factors also play a part, though their presence is less easy to determine, since the ways in which they may manifest themselves are more complex. The delight in logical thoroughness and systematization often represents a reaction-formation against the "productive" anal tendencies; the regular resort to certain rules of word-formation, etc., can moreover (as in Esperanto) make possible a great reduction in the *number* of root words, an achievement gratifying to the "retentive" anal tendencies, with which the above-mentioned reaction-formations would seem so often to co-operate. On the other hand, in actual practice, the endeavour to maintain logical consistency often leads to the use of longer words, which in turn is gratifying to the "productive" tendencies and is opposed by the reaction-formations thereto; while insistence on short words means an increase in the number of roots and an abandonment of system.

Under these conditions, conflicts between the various anal-erotic factors must assume a degree of complexity which it is scarcely possible to analyse without a more detailed study than can be here attempted.

We have arrived at the conclusion of our analysis, which, incomplete and fragmentary as it undoubtedly is, will at any rate, we may hope, serve to show that as dynamic factors underlying the international language movement are to be found certain unconscious

---

[1] The conflict between logical consistency and initial ease of understanding is in many (not all) respects the same as that between the two forms of language which historians of the international language movement have distinguished as *a priori* and *a posteriori* respectively.

mental mechanisms with which psycho-analysis has made us familiar. These unconscious mechanisms are, we have seen, themselves exceedingly complex in nature and in function. Not only do they belong to a variety of developmental levels (the allo-erotic, the genital auto-erotic [phallic] and the anal auto-erotic), but at each level there are ambivalencies prompting to behaviour in different, often in contrary, directions; the ultimate attitude of any individual towards the international language movement resulting thus from the interplay of many different factors, all of them normally outside the individual's power of intellectual appreciation or voluntary control. These mechanisms are, moreover, operative in one way or another, whatever be the relation of the individual to the movement; we have traced their influence in the inventors of international language, in leaders of propaganda, in the rank and file of those who adopt and use an international language, and in outsiders who merely come across the employment or advocacy of such a language.

Our investigation has also, as we anticipated, not been absolutely barren of results bearing on the wider psychological problems presented by language and by constructive social movements in general. It is clear that many of the factors which we have found operative in the international language movement are of a nature to affect the use of, and attitude towards, every kind of language (both "native" and "foreign"), while others of these factors are such as will be present also in social movements quite unconnected with linguistic matters. Our considerations have indeed, I venture to think, emphasized a point already fairly clear from previous work in applied psycho-analysis, namely, that the study of unconscious mental life may prove of the greatest service to the philologist and sociologist. Without daring overmuch, we may perhaps look forward to a period in the not too distant future when a knowledge of the deep-lying human motives revealed by psycho-analysts will be one of the most valuable possessions, both of those who would understand that most essential condition of our social life, the delicate mechanism by which ideas are communicated from one mind to another, and of those who seek to weigh the chances or control the course of actual social change or social progress.

ON THE SIGNIFICANCE OF NAMES[1]

By Ingeborg Flugel

It is perhaps surprising that so very little has been written on the psychological significance of names. Most people tend to think that beyond their obvious purpose of indicating or symbolizing persons, names can have at most only a historical or philological interest. And yet there can be little doubt that they have also a psychological aspect. Indeed, once this is pointed out, it immediately becomes apparent that names play a rôle of some importance in our mental life, and may even influence our conduct in subtle ways which we often fail to recognize. Few, if any, people are indifferent to names. It is an instructive experiment to ask a circle of friends to say which names they like and dislike, and to give as far as possible their reasons. One is then nearly always assured of some interesting information, for, superficially at any rate, names do not constitute an embarrassingly emotional topic, and most people are willing and able to talk about them, though they are often astonished at the discovery in themselves of preferences and emotional reactions, of the existence and reasons of which they had before been unaware.

It has long been recognized that the names of characters in fiction have some considerable importance for our appreciation of the qualities and motives of the individuals portrayed, and that great novelists may possess a special ability for the selection of appropriate

[1] Reprinted from *The British Journal of Medical Psychology*, 1930.

designations. Zola even went so far as to condemn offhand an author who appeared to lack this skill. "I am quite a fatalist," he wrote, "in the matter of names, believing firmly that a mysterious correlation exists between the man and the name he bears. Thus I always judge a young author by the names which he bestows upon his characters. If the names seem to be weak or to be unsuitable to the people who bear them, I put the author down as a man of little talent, and am no further interested in his book."[1]

A definitely psychological interest in the subject of names seems to date from the period immediately preceding the Great War. Professor Weekley in his book on *The Romance of Names*, though treating the subject principally from a philological aspect,[2] nevertheless points out that "Bull" and "Muddiman" are singularly appropriate names for Rugby footballers; and, in view of some remarks relative to himself, he would probably admit that the peculiarities of his own name have not been without effect on his interest on the subject of names in general.

Following on some experiments of Kollarits,[3] Claparède[4] suggested that a name tends to call up the image of a person of a definite type and that this type is more or less constant for all who hear the name, *e.g.* that names with heavy or repeated syllables make us think of fat, thick-set or bloated individuals, that a short name suggests a slim and active person, and so on. Thus Monsieur Patapoufard would be of a different

---

[1] E. Zola. Introduction to *Dr. Pascal*.

[2] Ernest Weekley. *The Romance of Names*, 1913, pp. 2, 27.

[3] J. Kollarits. "Observations de Psychologie Quotidienne," *Archives de Psychologie*, 1914, XIV, p. 225.

[4] E. Claparède. "Sur la Représentation des Personnes Inconnues." *Archives de Psychologie*, 1914, XIV, p. 301.

type to Monsieur Flic. English,[1] however, while corroborating the general associative significance of names, found that individuals differ greatly in their interpretation of any given name.

Alspach,[2] with the help of a long list of quaint imaginary names, found that their associative significance depended upon such factors as nationality, known persons of similar name, auditory-verbal associations (as when Gronch suggested grouch and grunt), and the sound of the word (as when in Snemth Sn appears as "a mean sound" and the shortness of the word seems to indicate lack of respect).

Gordon[3] and de Laski[4] studied the methods by which Charles Dickens arrived at his proper names and showed that all the above-mentioned factors played a part in the process.

Several psycho-analytic writers had, however, already approached the subject from their own point of view. Stekel[5] was the first of this school to draw attention to the often unconscious significance of names in determining conduct and emotional attitude, while Rank and Abraham soon afterwards brought forward further evidence in that direction.[6]

[1] G. English. "On the Psychological Response to Proper Names," *American Journal of Psychology*, 1916, XXV, p. 417.

[2] E. M. Alspach. "On the Psychological Response to Unknown Proper Names," *American Journal of Psychology*, 1917, XXVIII, p. 436.

[3] E. H. Gordon. "The Naming of Characters in the Works of Charles Dickens," *University of Nebraska, Studies in Language, Literature and Criticism*, 1917.

[4] E. de Laski. "The Psychological Attitude of Charles Dickens towards Surnames," *American Journal of Psychology*, 1918, XXIX, p. 337.

[5] Wilhelm Stekel. "Die Verpflichtung des Namens," *Zeitschrift für Psychotherapie und Medizinische Psychologie*, III, Heft 2, 1911.

[6] Otto Rank. *Das Inzestmotiv in Dichtung und Sage*, 1912, p. 93, footnote; Karl Abraham, "Über die determinierende Kräfte des Namens," *Centralblatt für Psychoanalyse*, 1912, II, p. 133.

The cases of unconscious influence of name on conduct that have been observed by myself, seem to fall naturally into three main divisions (though with more extended research further categories may become desirable): (1) general influence on character and behaviour, (2) choice of profession or occupation, (3) choice of love object—though in certain cases the influence of a name may manifest itself in more than one of these categories.

With regard to the first category, Christ was clearly alive to the influence of names on character when he said "Thou art Peter, and upon this rock (πέτρος) I will build my church."[1] Here we have an assumption of an effect on both character and future occupation.

In other cases, the influence of name on character may reveal itself largely through the love-life of the individual.   Benjamin Constant, in his little *chef d'œuvre, Adolphe*, makes the hero remain "constant" to his mistress through countless difficulties, and this story, as Sainte-Beuve informs us, combines "*art et verité.*" Sometimes, however, names have certainly a contra-suggestive effect; the person refuses to take the character his name indicates, and develops rather the opposite qualities. To give two examples. A girl, known to me, and called "Desirée" (after, as she put it, "a sainted aunt"), from her earliest childhood hated and rebelled against her name. "It soured my whole life and I just tried to become as undesirable as possible." In this case, we have a combined effect of the *meaning* of a name and its *association* with a particular person. It represents, therefore, a transition to that other type of case, in which a person hates his name purely on account of its associations; as in the example described

---

[1] Matthew xvi, 18.

by Stekel[1] in which a girl suffered from a disability to use or mention her surname, because of the shortcomings of her father. Another case of contra-suggestive influence is that of a man whose Christian name is "Lord," and who, in spite of ample opportunity to lead a life of aristocratic ease, both practises and preaches the most democratic principles; though it is true that a slight ambivalence shows itself in certain aspects of his life—in particular, he took a wife whose (foreign) Christian name had the etymological significance of "Lady."

The influence of name on *profession* can scarcely be doubted, though, in view of the difficulty of estimating the likelihood of mere chance combinations between name and profession, it is desirable to lay stress only on cases where the combination is particularly striking, or unlikely to occur by chance, or where one has definite information that the name did in fact exercise an influence. As Abraham[2] points out, Goethe had already recognized the possibility of an influence of this sort in his description of a man named Mittler,[3] who made it his business to act as a "Mediator" between those who quarrelled. About the same time Karl Philipp Moritz, in his "psychological novel," *Anton Reiser*, recognizes the same mechanism when he describes his hero's departure for Bremen with the words: "This was the first strange romantic journey which Anton Reiser took, and from this time forward he began to justify his name (*Reiser* – traveller [*sic*])."[4]

It may be that names often exercise, so to speak, a

---

[1] Wilhelm Stekel. "Warum sie den eigenen Namen hassen," *Centralblatt für Psychoanalyse*, 1911 I, p. 109.

[2] Karl Abraham, *loc. cit.*

[3] Goethe, *Wahlverwandtschaften*, Pt. I, chap. ii.

[4] Translated by P. E. Matheson, Oxford University Press, p. 297.

quantitative as well as a qualitative effect on character, that is, they may increase or diminish the amount of "drive" possessed by an individual, as well as determine the direction of his "drive." Some recent evidence from China points in this direction. In a research by T. Y. Lo,[1] in which some seven hundred names selected from a biographical directory were estimated according to degree of fame, it was found that the more famous men more frequently possessed meaningful names than did the less famous. When the results were classified into two big groups, 60 per cent. of the more famous, and only 28 per cent. of the less famous had meaningful names. If we can generalize from this, it would seem that the possession of a name with *any* kind of meaning tends to develop those character-qualities that lead to prominence, and that those whose names appear to be arbitrary symbols without further significance are at a disadvantage in the race of life.

Coming to the more definite professions, numerous examples could be cited from the most varied fields; Sonne is a well-known authority on the medical application of artificial sunlight, Hare is the author of a book on premature whitening of the hair, Landon is an estate agent, Hilda Glyder is a dancer, Utteridge is "the man with the golden voice," Henry Hyde sells boots and shoes, Eben. E. Fowler has a bird and cage depôt, J. P. Draper advertises "superior shirts and collars," Lightfoot is a professional skater, Pfeifer (Piper) is a psycho-analyst whose written works deal chiefly with the psychology of music, Walter Chain is appropriately enough a sanitary engineer, Cutbush

[1] T. Y. Lo, " Correlation of name and fame," *Chinese J. of Psychol.*, 1925, III.

is recognized as the greatest authority on topiary work in England. In some cases, however, a person may refuse from self-consciousness or embarrassment to adopt a profession indicated by his name; I have heard of a butcher who had some repugnance to this profession, and so became a baker—"as the next best thing." In other cases, however, the attraction of a name-indicated profession may overcome many obstacles. Recently in Germany, I came across a Cupferschmid (Coppersmith) whose father kept a garage, and who in spite of a good opening here, left to become a coppersmith—though afterwards he was reluctantly compelled for financial reasons to return to the motor business. In view of examples like these, which could be multiplied, it seems quite possible that a person's name may often have had some influence in dictating interests, even where the occupation has a less obvious connection with the meaning of the name. Thus, to become bolder, it may be no chance that it was just a Mr. Pullman who invented an improved method of transporting his fellow-men, and that Richard Ungewitter (bad weather) so reconciled himself to the inclemencies of climate as to preach and practise nudity even in the snows.

Turning now to the effect of name on *choice of love object*, we find that fixation is on the whole more important than meaning. Nevertheless meaning is an influence in certain cases as, for instance, in the pretty example recently described by Professor Nunn[1] of the Greek poet Philodemus, who fell in love with four Demo's in succession and definitely recognized that his name had determined his fate as a lover. An author

[1] Sir T. Percy Nunn, " The Fatal Name," *International Journal of Psycho-Analysis*, 1929, X, p. 97.

of more recent times, whose several heroines are all of masterful and violent dispositions, married a Miss Rough. The significance of names can, moreover, scarcely be absent in the case of a lady who married in succession a Mr. Merriman and a Mr. Glad.

The influence of fixation in determining a succession of love objects is clearly shown in several great poets. The case of Schiller's three Charlottes—Charlotte von Wolzogen, Charlotte von Kalb, Charlotte von Lengefeld—and that of Shelley's three Harriets—Harriet Grove, Harriet Westbrook, and Harriet de Boinville—are fairly well known, having already been mentioned by several authors in this connection. Byron was in his own words "utterly devotedly fond" of Mary Duff when he was barely eight, and thereafter had innumerable attachments to women bearing the name of Mary, Marion, etc., as many of his poems bear witness. He was undoubtedly justified when he wrote:

> I have a passion for the name of Mary,
> For once it was a magic sound to me:
> And still it half calls up the realms of fairy,
> Where I beheld what never was to be:
> All feelings change, but this was last to vary,
> A spell from which even yet I am not free.[1]

From my own observations it appears to me that the name of "Mary" (together with its derivatives) exercises something like a universal attraction on men. It is a name closely connected by clang association (and perhaps, too, in the last resort etymologically) with words for mother and words for sea (itself one of the most universal mother symbols; cf. *la Mer*, *la Mère*). The root *Ma* (in Sanskrit = to produce), with the meaning of mother, is itself one of the earliest forms

---

[1] Byron, *Don Juan*, 7.

of speech in the development of the individual throughout the globe[1] and, as Spielrein has suggested,[2] may
be derived from the act of sucking. But the fascination
of the name is tempered by taboo, especially since in
Christian countries Mary, the Immaculate and semi-
divine mother, sheds some of her chaste glory on all
her namesakes. Owing to such a taboo on an early
(usually incestuous) love, it sometimes happens that
subsequent attachments are formed towards persons
whose name merely resembles that of the original love
object. Thus, in one case, an only son, who had long
lived with his mother Elizabeth, was greatly attracted
by the name Betty. Another man, whose sister was
called Dorothy, from early youth upwards has repeatedly
fallen in love with women called Doreen or Doris.
Sometimes the resemblance, without being less striking,
is a little less direct, as in a case known to me, where a
man whose mother's maiden name was Anerley,
married an Anna Lee, and in announcing his engagement told his friends: "she is as beautiful as her name."

Little attention has hitherto been paid to the reasons
for giving names to children. It is usually assumed,
doubtless correctly, that family tradition is the most
important factor here. Nevertheless, a study of these
cases where there is a departure from this tradition
would probably be very instructive. In one instance
known to me, a mother selected for her child the Latin
name of a flower, and the choice was shown by subsequent free association to be determined largely by
the fact that she had first learnt of this name from her
father (an ardent botanist). The giving of the name

---

[1] Cf. Jespersen, *Language*, p. 154.
[2] Spielrein, "Die Entstehung der kindlichen Worte Papa und Mama,"
Imago, 1922, VIII, p. 345.

to her child signified to the unconscious that she had received the child (as she had actually received the name) from her father. In many cases, of course, children are named after famous persons, who presumably correspond to certain ideals of the parents. It seems to be generally assumed that such names have an effect upon the ideals of the child. At any rate, the only case I know in which a Government interfered with the christening of a child, was in the case of the Swiss Government, which refused to allow a child to be called "Trotsky," lest revolutionary aspirations should be instilled into him at his very birth.

We have the privilege of naming not only the children of our bodies, but also those of our imagination; novelists in particular (to return to a matter on which we have already touched) can exercise their fancy in giving names to their characters, and it is certain that many of the instances quoted could be paralleled from fiction. Here the mention of one example must suffice: the heroines of the popular French author, Pierre Benoit, begin nearly always with the letter A—Atlantide, Axelle, Aurore, Alice, Alberte, Agar, etc. I have no private information as to the cause of this similarity, but, in view especially of the fact that they have also certain character qualities in common, it is almost impossible not to suppose that in his successive heroines the author has, as it were, created so many reincarnations of an original love object. Kings have certain privileges not granted to ordinary mortals; and King Ludwig II of Bavaria, among his other eccentricities, insisted upon altering the name of his fiancée (to whom he was unwillingly betrothed and whom he never married) from Sophie to Elsa, under the influence of the heroine of Wagner's *Lohengrin* and—it is rumoured—of an affection for the Empress Elizabeth of Austria.   In this way an attempt was perhaps made to give some semblance of charm to an otherwise unattractive matrimonial prospect.

I am well aware that in this short article I have left many aspects untouched.   Many further examples of the kind I have quoted will occur to everybody.   I have here endeavoured to do little more than merely draw attention to a fascinating field of research, that is far from having been as yet exhausted.

SOME PSYCHOLOGICAL ASPECTS OF A FOX-HUNTING RITE[1]

By Ingeborg Flugel

THERE is practised in England to-day a curious hunting rite, which is well known to all followers of hounds, but which, perhaps because of its very strangeness and barbarity, is seldom, if ever, mentioned in the copious literature of hunting. When a person—nowadays usually a child—is present at a kill of a fox for the first time,[2] the Master, taking some severed portion of the animal, smears some of the blood upon the face of the person, who is not allowed to wash it off until the evening. This procedure of "Blooding" or "Christening," as it is called, is regarded as an honour, and, to judge from various accounts I have collected, usually gives great pleasure to the parents of the children who are blooded, though the children themselves naturally react to the ceremony very varyingly. Some are not a little terrified. One small boy cried bitterly, until, to the dismay of his parents (who belonged to a well-known fox-hunting family) it became necessary to wash the blood-stains away before the appointed time. Others are proud of the distinction; indeed, the late H. W. Selby-Lowndes, who was blooded at four and a half, refused to have his face washed even at bedtime.[3] What can be the meaning

---

[1] Reprinted from the *International Journal of Psycho-Analysis*, 1931, XII.
[2] The same rite is sometimes practised in hare and otter hunting.
[3] *Hunting Reminiscences* of H. W. Selby-Lowndes.

of this curious and bloody rite which, if reported of a primitive people, would surely be regarded as a sign of savagery? It is clear we have to do here with an initiation ceremony. Indeed, in the words of a recent correspondent,[1] "the boy or girl who has been blooded, is definitely considered to be admitted to the ranks of Nimrod and Diana." To be blooded is, as we have said, an honour—a point which it has in common with all initiation ceremonies. But we have to ask why the honour should take this peculiar form. There can be very little doubt that the smearing with the fox's blood indicates that the initiated has himself participated in the kill, and thus shared both the honour and the guilt attaching to the deed. He has become one of those to whom Mark Antony refers:[2]

> . . . 'And here thy hunters stand
> Signed in thy spoil, and crimsoned in thy lethe.'

To realize the full meaning of this honour, we must pass from fox-hunting to other forms of hunting which preceded it. In the earlier days, it was indeed esteemed a special honour actually to kill the hunted animal when brought to bay, and only those of a certain social standing were allowed this privilege—a privilege which, it was dimly supposed, was not unappreciated by the animal itself, for there seems little doubt that some genuine feeling finds expression by the mocking words of A. P. Herbert, when he says in *Tantivy Towers*:—

> And one of the jolliest features
>   Of slaying superfluous game
> Is the thought that we're saving the creatures
>   From a death of dishonour and shame—

---

[1] R. J. Fairfax-Blakeborough : *Notes and Queries*, March 8th, 1930.
[2] *Julius Cæsar*, III, i, 204.

And they're lucky to die as they do,
  For if they do not
They're sure to be shot
  By someone who's not in *Who's Who*.
And I give you my word
  That a sensitive bird—
A point for our foolish reproachers—
  Prefers its career
To be stopped by a peer
  And not by unmannerly poachers.

The animal could only be killed or cut up in a certain way, by certain instruments, or after certain ceremonies. Erasmus[1] writing at the beginning of the sixteenth century says: "When they have run down their game, what strange pleasure they take in cutting it up; cows and sheep may be slaughtered by common butchers, but what is killed in hunting must be broke up by none under a gentleman, who shall throw down his hat, fall devoutly on his knees, and, drawing out a slashing hanger (for a common knife is not good enough), after several ceremonies, shall dissect all the parts as artificially as the best skilled anatomist, while all that stand around shall look very intently." There exists for instance a contemporary picture of a kneeling huntsman offering to Queen Elizabeth a knife with which to cut the throat of a stag which is lying on his back before her. But it would seem that other noble dames had sometimes the same privilege, for Pope[2] refers to the compliment our huntsmen pass on ladies of quality, who are present. at the death of a stag, when they put a knife in their hands to cut its throat, a custom which he describes as "barbarous enough to be derived from the Goths or even the Scythians." The fact that it is regarded as a special honour to be allowed to kill the hunted animal

---

[1] Erasmus : *Morias Encomion.*   [2] Pope : *Guardian*, No. 61.

is in harmony with the general attitude towards hunting as a whole, which was considered an aristocratic pastime, the mere participation in which was to some extent a privilege. Poaching has always been regarded as a serious offence, often punished with a severity quite out of proportion to the material damage that was done. This applied particularly to any attempt to hunt or chase animals belonging to the King, against which crime the laws demanded that the most terrible penalties should be inflicted. In England "the earliest forest laws of which there is record are those of Canute (1016). Under these, if a freeman offered violence to a keeper of the King's deer he was liable to lose freedom and prosperity; if a serf, he lost his right hand, and on a second offence, was to die. One who killed a deer, was either to have his eyes put out or to lose his life. Under the first two Norman kings, mutilation was the punishment for poaching."[1] It is true that in England, fox-hunting has been democratized for 150 years at least, but traces of special privilege still remain. One cannot ask to be "blooded"; it is a compliment that must be freely offered, and the same applies to special colours and hunt insignia—no one may wear these insignia unless asked to by the Master, whose offer has the force of a command, for at the next meeting of the hunt, colours, buttons, etc., must all be in order.

But, though hunting itself was a privilege, those who enjoyed this privilege had nevertheless to observe most punctiliously the ritual of the sport, a ritual which culminated in the act of killing, dissecting and distributing the quarry, and according to which certain specially valued parts (mask, brush, pads, etc., in the case of foxes) were allotted to some particularly honoured

[1] *Encyclopædia Britannica*, 11th Edition. Article on " Mutilation."

persons, and the rest thrown to the hounds as their share of the spoil. Now this ritual would seem to imply that the hunted animal itself was honoured: a conclusion which emerges both from hunting literature and the ritual itself. As an example from more modern literature let us quote Whyte-Melville [1] as regards the stag: "But of all the forest creatures hunted by our forefathers and ourselves, the stag has been considered from time immemorial the noblest beast of chase. His nature had been the study of princes, his pursuit the sport of kings. The education of royalty would have been thought incomplete without a thorough knowledge of his haunts and habits, while books were written and authorities quoted on the formalities with which his courteous persecutors deemed it becoming that he should be hunted to death . . . an animal that can fly twenty miles on end for life, and die with its back to the rock, undaunted in defeat, a true gentleman to the last, is surely no unworthy object of pursuit." [2]

With regard to the ritual we may refer once more to Erasmus' description of the "gentleman" who "shall throw down his hat" and "fall devoutly on his knees before despatching the game." Such extreme signs of respect as are here indicated surely give the clue to the whole attitude involved in these ceremonies. They overwhelmingly suggest a religious sacrifice — an institution, the most primitive and the

---

[1] *Katerfelto*, p. 214.

[2] The facts that the hunted animal itself was held in honour, and that the killing of it was a princely privilege, are both well brought out in the continuation of the already quoted passage from *Julius Cæsar* :—

> " O World ! Thou wast the forest to this hart ;
> And this indeed, O World ! the heart of thee.
> How like a deer stricken by many princes,
> Dost thou here lie : "

clearest examples of which are to be found in the ritual of totemism. If the attitude of the hunter in modern Europe really retains some totemic elements we should expect to find a parallelism in other details also.

Traces of such a parallelism are indeed not wanting. We know, for instance, that the attitude of the clansman towards his totem is distinctly ambivalent,[1] a fluctuating medley of veneration, fear, hatred, and even of friendliness. The fox is to some extent the recipient of all these feelings. The hunter's attitude towards him differs markedly according to the seasons. As the famous Mr. Jorrocks says in Surtees' *Handley Cross*, . . . "In the summer I loves him with the hardour of affection, not an 'air of his beautiful 'ead would I hurt: the sight of him is more glorious nor the Lord Mayor's show! but when the hautumn comes—when the brownin' copse and cracklin' stubble proclaim the farmers' fears are past, then, dash my vig, 'ow I glories in pursuing him to distruction, and holding him above the bayin' pack." A similar ambivalence, but one that is more stable in its manifestations, is shown by those who, from being keen fox-hunters, subsequently become active opponents of the sport. At the present time the hostility to "Blood Sports" would seem to be gaining ground in some quarters. At any rate this school of thought recently captured a majority at a meeting of the "Dumb Friends' League," an event which led to the resignation of the then President, Lord Lonsdale. Perhaps the earliest recorded instance of the change of attitude in question, is that of St. Hubert, who, according to the well-known tradition, desisted from hunting after an occasion on which he had seen a stag with a luminous crucifix miraculously suspended be-

[1] Freud : *Totem and Taboo.*

tween its horns. As this incident which brought about
the saint's conversion happened on a Good Friday, there
seems little doubt that the hunted animal was unconsciously identified with the crucified Saviour Himself—
a fact which once again reveals the deicidal (*i.e.* in the
last resort totemic) element in hunting. The continuance
of the ambivalent attitude in later generations is, moreover, manifested by the fact that St. Hubert has been
made the patron saint of hunters, in spite of the fact
that his canonization is connected, not with his prosecution, but with his abandonment, of hunting.

The honour and respect shown to the fox (as to other
hunted animals) accords ill with the cruel manner of
his death—a common feature of totemism and of the
corresponding sacrifices of divine persons or animals
in the higher religions. Ambivalence is shown even
in the disposal of the remains ; for while certain parts,
such as the mask, brush and pads,[1] are highly valued,
and are themselves only presented to honoured persons,
the remaining portions are thrown ignominiously
to the hounds — an act which, if we can trust the
linguistic parallel of "going to the dogs," certainly
implies contempt. The numerous stories illustrating
the proverbial cleverness of the fox show that we see
in him a creature of fantastic cunning,[2] but almost
always with evil intent—in short, the nearest approach
to an incarnation of the devil in animal form. It is not
perhaps surprising to read in *The Gentlemen's Recreation*
of *circa* 1650[3] that: 'if greyhounds course him on a
plain, his last refuge is to piss on his tail, and to flop it

[1] The tail of the fox can of course be a phallic symbol, as was recognized
by Gubernatis. (Fowler : *Roman Festivals*).

[2] As illustrated, for instance, in the greatest of all fox epics, Goethe's
Reinecke Fuchs.

[3] N. Cox : *The Gentlemen's Recreation*.

on their faces, sometimes squirting his thicker excrement upon them to make them give over the course of pursuit." But we may open our eyes when we find the following account of his almost incredible ingenuity in the latest edition of the *Encyclopædia Britannica*: "Taking in his mouth a tuft of wool, or a piece of wood, a fox will slowly sink himself, tail first, into a pond, and thus gradually drive the fleas forward until their last refuge is on the wood or wool on the surface of the water. The fox then sets this adrift teeming with the parasites, and, keeping clear of it, lands on the bank and makes off."

Another parallel with the totemic animal is that the fox can be killed only in certain ways and in certain seasons, as a collective deed performed with the due ritual. To shoot a fox in modern England is almost as wicked as for a member of a totemic community to kill his totem otherwise than in the appointed manner. As a hunting friend said to me concerning the fox shooter, "his name is less than mud"; and the curse pronounced upon such persons in that exquisite document, *The Fox Hunter's Creed*, dedicated to Selby-Lowndes by T. C. Young, ex-M.F.H. of Haydon hounds, has the true smack of primitive magic: "He that killeth or taketh a fox by any means save by hunting, let him be accursed. Yea, let him be everlastingly damned, may his dwelling become desolate, and his possessions a desert; may his soul be filled with bitterness, and his body with pain."

Another important feature of totemism is that the clansman to some extent identifies himself with the totem by means of sacrifice. In this sacrifice, identification usually takes place by eating, through which the divine essence is incorporated in each participant. An

ambivalent attitude is shown here by the fact that the
holy meal is usually preceded by a fast.   Faint relics
of feasting and fasting are to be seen in connection with
hunting also.   At least, we can read in another article
of *The Fox Hunter's Creed*, this time in distinctly
religious phraseology: " If it be possible let every true
believer of the faith abstain from all food and drink
during the day, save only sufficient to sustain life in
case of need.   The whole day is to be spent as a special
fasting, and strengthening of the mind in the Faith.
He shall partake of food and drink in the evening.
Verily after a good day he shall partake of a special
allowance of drink."   This is clearly reminiscent of the
ritual of fasting that so often precedes both the eating
of the totem and the equivalent ceremonies in the more
developed religions, not excluding that of the Christian
Communion service.[1]   It may be that the practice of
"blooding" or "christening" (a term borrowed from the
first ceremony of initiation into the church) which to
some extent establishes a physical connection or identity,
between initiate and fox, springs from motives that are
not altogether dissimilar from those that impel the
worshipper to seek identity with the divine victim.   At
any rate in Borneo the killing of an animal corresponding
to an individual totem may be accompanied by sacrifice
in which blood is smeared upon the sacrificer.[2]   The
smearing of blood upon the face may even be a shortened

[1] The ambivalent attitude in the Communion service is revealed by the
doctrine that, whereas participation in the Communion is highly beneficial
to the pious, it is full of danger if we partake of it unworthily, for then " we
are guilty of the body and blood of Christ, Our Saviour [*i.e.* become His
murderers] and drink our own damnation ; not considering the Lord's body,
we kindle God's wrath against us, we provoke Him to plague us with divers
diseases, and sundry kinds of death."   It is clear that the old feelings of
guilt connected with sacrifice are not so very deeply buried.

[2] Frazer, *Totemism and Exogamy*, II, pp. 210, 211.

and symbolic expression of the more primitive practice of drinking the blood; for in certain initiation ceremonies of Australian tribes the initiates are covered with the blood of fellow-tribesmen, which at the same time they drink;[1] the meaning of this covering with blood in the sense of identification being, in Frazer's opinion, "beyond a doubt."

Another parallel between the totemic sacrifice and hunting is the desire in both cases that all present shall continue to participate until the end of the ceremony —a desire that, in the case of sacrifice, undoubtedly springs, not only from the wish that all should share the benefits, but partly also from the need to share the guilt. It was for this reason that we suggested earlier that "blooding" might also constitute a sign of partnership in guilt. At any rate the author of *The Fox Hunter's Creed* disapproves highly of anyone desisting from the hunt before the end, for another of his articles ran: "accursed be he that goeth home of his own free will before hounds." Corresponding to the elaborate ceremonial in the case both of hunting and of totemic sacrifice is the need for special instruction for those who are to become initiated. The explanation of totemic ceremonies constitutes an important part of the initiation ceremonies of primitive peoples. As regards hunting we have already heard that the education of royalty itself was deemed incomplete without a thorough knowledge of the chase, and of the "haunts and habits" of the hunted animals. In *The Fox Hunter's Creed*, moreover, we read: "It is lawful and right that those of experience shall carefully give explanation and encouragement to all young persons and instruct by word and deed at all times, so that

---

[1] *Op. cit.*, I, p. 42 ; IV, p. 200.

fox-hunting shall continue in the land from generation to generation. He that thinketh he knoweth, but knoweth not, let him be accursed."

Finally, we may note that, just as in certain religions containing totemic elements, the sacrifice of an animal and of a human being can be regarded with very similar feelings, so too in hunting, there are not wanting traces of an association between the slaying of the hunted animal and the death of a man. There exists a tradition that the ceremony of cutting off the right foot of a stag and presenting it to the most honoured guest owes its origin to the old feudal right known as "main morte," by which a seigneur, "had the right hand of any of his serfs who died brought to him as an indisputable proof that the serf in question was in all truth defunct and had not feigned death and fled, in the hopes of obtaining his freedom."[1] But the practice of "main morte" was itself almost certainly merely an adaptation of the more primitive and widespread custom of cutting off the hands or otherwise mutilating enemies killed in war. A most dramatic example of the association between killing of a hunted stag and an attempted murder of a rival, is to be found in Whyte-Melville's already quoted novel *Katerfelto*, in which the villain attempts to kill the hero at the very moment when the latter is dispatching the stag. That this is no chance association is shown by the villain's previous musings when contemplating his rival's downfall: "How much better," he thought, "to track him as Tancred (a favourite hound) tracked the deer, never slacking in effort, never off the scent, never turning aside for any consideration, till he had run him ruthlessly down."

Though the resemblance between totemism and

---

[1] W. A. Baillie-Grohman : *Sport in Art*, 2nd Ed., p. 330.

hunting, as regards any one of the points we have mentioned, may perhaps seem to depend on somewhat slender evidence, the correspondence as a whole is nevertheless worthy of consideration. No one, I think, can deny that hunting appeals to primitive instincts, and a kill seems necessary to the full enjoyment. If we are right in assuming that the kill awakens faint echoes of deep totemic tendencies, the satisfaction that it so universally affords is perhaps made somewhat clearer, and we can understand better the profound content that the successful sportsman manifests. We can see, too, perhaps, why hunting continues to be popular (for some hunts to-day are in danger of being overcrowded) even — as at the present time — after the bloodiest of wars, when it might have been supposed that there had been enough of killing. Finally, we can understand why there is a tendency for the hunted animal, whatever it may be, to be regarded with esteem, and to be honoured by a certain ritual. Foxes, formerly looked upon as vermin, have now become the recipients of feelings that formerly, and more naturally, were directed to the stag, which has now almost ceased to be available. It seems not impossible that some day, for a similar reason, we may have the same feelings towards the humble rabbit.

So by tortuous ways, aided by the versatility of human nature, does man continue to fulfil his deepest tendencies.

ON THE CHARACTER AND MARRIED LIFE
OF HENRY VIII[1]

IT is doubtful whether the married life of any monarch
in the world's history has aroused such interest and
attained such notoriety as that of Henry VIII. In
popular estimation the relations of King Henry to his
wives probably outweigh in fascination all other
features of a lengthy and momentous reign; while
even to the professed historian the study of Henry's
six marriages—closely connected as they are with
events of great significance occurring at a particularly
critical period in the cultural and political development
of Europe—must also be of very considerable importance. No apology is needed therefore for attempting a further treatment of this theme—even in brief
and summary fashion—if by so doing we can throw a
few fresh rays of light upon the factors which were at
work in producing the events recorded in this page of
history.

A well-known historian, commenting on the long
series of Henry's matrimonial experiences, has justly
remarked that "a single misadventure of such a kind
might have been explained by accident or by moral
infirmity. For such a combination of disasters some
common cause must have existed, which may be, or
ought to be, discoverable."[2] It has seemed to the

---

[1] Reprinted from *The International Journal of Psycho-Analysis*, 1920,
Vol. I.

[2] J. A. Froude, *History of England*, II, p. 469.

present writer that the common cause in question is to be found largely in certain constant features of Henry's mental life and character, the proper understanding of which concerns the psychologist as much as the historian. It is in the hope of indicating the nature of some of the more important of these constant features that the present essay has been written. The conclusions at which it arrives are tentative only, and are put forward with all the diffidence that is due to the circumstance that the writer is very well aware of the shortcomings of his historical knowledge and training. The historical materials bearing on the reign of Henry VIII are very numerous and would require years of patient study for their adequate assimilation: indeed it is evident that their complete elucidation and evaluation at the hands of historians are as yet far from having been accomplished. Much that is here suggested may therefore have to be revised, both as the result of expert historical criticism and of an increased understanding of the relevant facts. The application of psychological knowledge to the task of interpreting the events of history will, however, certainly constitute a very necessary piece of work for future scholarship, and as a small addition to the relatively few attempts that have been made in this direction, the following suggestions as to the nature of the psychological influences at work in the married life of Henry VIII may perhaps be of some interest both to psychologists and to historians.

It is unfortunate that, in spite of the many known facts which bear upon the adult life of Henry VIII, our knowledge of his early life is very slender. The researches of Freud and the workers of his school have shown that a knowledge of the events of childhood and of youth is a very valuable aid to the interpretation of the mental characteristics of later years. In the case of Henry VIII, however, we have to be content with few facts and these mostly connected with affairs of state but little calculated to throw light on questions of psychology.

Henry was born in June, 1491, and was the fourth of his parents' five children, the earlier children being Arthur (Henry's only brother), Margaret (afterwards Queen of Scotland), and Elizabeth (who died in infancy), while the single younger child was Mary (afterwards Queen of France and, later, Duchess of Suffolk). Henry's father (Henry VII) had ascended the throne of England as the result of his triumph over Richard III in the last battle of the War of the Roses, and by his able and successful rule of twenty-four years had definitely put an end to that bloody and disastrous struggle. He had claimed the throne by right of inheritance and conquest; but to add to the strength of his position he had married Elizabeth of York, eldest daughter of Edward IV, uniting thus the rival houses whose dissensions had devastated England for the preceding thirty years. There was indeed a difficulty in the match, inasmuch as Henry and Elizabeth were within the prohibited degrees of affinity (both being descended from Catherine, wife of Henry V), a papal dispensation being necessary before the marriage could legally be made. Henry, however, anxious no doubt for the additional security of title which the marriage would provide, did not wait to receive the dispensation, and the wedding was celebrated a few months after he ascended the throne—the dispensation fortunately arriving shortly afterwards.

Throughout the reign there were not wanting efforts

of rival claimants to the throne to displace Henry from the position he had won, nor uprisings on the part of a people grown ill used to settled government. The long conflict between the rival Roses did not give place suddenly to an era of assured internal peace, but, in dying, continued for many years to manifest itself in minor upheavals which formed a continual menace to the sovereignty of the first of the Tudors. Henry, it is true, successfully weathered every storm that threatened to engulf him, and was in the main upheld by the great majority of his subjects, who realized that his rule was the only alternative to a return of anarchy and civil war. Nevertheless, we cannot but suppose that the difficulties and dangers which surrounded his father's throne must have exercised a powerful influence over the younger Henry's mind. The envy with which, even in ordinary families, a son is apt to look upon the superior powers and privileges of a father, is liable to be intensified when the father enjoys the exceptional influence and honour appertaining to a king. Under these circumstances any threat to the father's authority almost inevitably arouses in the son the idea of superseding the father.

In the present case such ideas were liable to be still further reinforced by the following facts:—first, that the mother's claim to the throne (and therefore of course that of her children) was regarded by confirmed Yorkists as superior to that of the father; and, secondly, that the marriage of the parents was not a happy one; the behaviour of the elder Henry being in general much wanting in warmth and affection towards his consort, in spite of the good looks, piety and learning by which the latter is reported to have been distinguished.

The conditions were thus favourable: (1) for the

arousal in young Henry's mind of the hope and desire to succeed to his father's place of authority (tendencies which may have been still further strengthened by the fact that he was invested at a tender age with various high offices—a device of his father's for concentrating as much power as possible in his own hands); (2) for the development of a powerful Œdipus complex, *i.e.* the desire to get rid of the father and possess the mother in his stead—the cold relations between mother and father and the beauty and goodness of the mother both constituting strong incentives to that desire.

The hostile feelings towards the father which may well have arisen under these circumstances were, however, in the case of young Prince Henry, fated to suffer to a large extent a process of displacement on to the person of his elder brother Arthur. To ambitious younger sons the privileges of primogeniture are always irksome; particularly so, it would seem, in the case of royal families, where the privileges in question are so exceptional in nature. In the present case young Henry's title to succeed his father was of course barred by the presence of Arthur—a prince who seems to have possessed qualities and abilities not inferior to those of his younger brother, and whose future reign was destined, in the hopes of many persons, to mark the opening of a new period of peace and prosperity, free from the unhappy dissensions of the immediate past.[1]

In 1501, when Henry was ten years old, Arthur, himself then only just fifteen, was married to Catherine

[1] This hope was indicated in the very choice of the name of the young Prince of Wales—a name which aroused no painful or exciting memories of the period of civil war, but which was associated with noble traditions of remoter British history.

Q

of Aragon, daughter of Ferdinand of Aragon and Isabella of Castile. Henry was no mere spectator at the wedding ceremony, but led his sister-in-law and future wife to the altar. At her formal reception into England, six weeks earlier, he had already played an equally important part. It is not improbable that these events induced in Henry some degree of jealousy towards his brother, thus adding a sexual element to the more purely personal envy which may well already have existed. To meet a comely girl and to hand her over with much ceremony to a brother—a brother who already appears to possess more than a fair share of the good things of life—is a procedure which is well calculated to arouse an emotion of this kind. Students of folklore and legend are familiar with the not infrequent type of story in which a situation of this sort is represented—the young hero being dispatched to welcome, and escort to her new home, the bride destined for the prince or king—stories which usually end with the awakening of illicit love between the hero and the lady, whose hand is already promised to another. In the light of later events we may perhaps be permitted to suppose that Henry, in spite of his youth, did not altogether escape the temptations to which his legendary predecessors in the same office had succumbed, and that the sexual elements of the Œdipus complex (which, as we know, are present in every child, and which, as is abundantly clear to the psycho-analyst, find expression in the legends in question) received in this way an additional motive for the transference on to brother and sister-in-law respectively of the feelings originally directed on to father and mother.

Arthur and Catherine had but little time in which

to enjoy their married life. For a few months they kept a merry court as Prince and Princess of Wales at Ludlow Castle, and then Arthur succumbed to an attack of the sweating sickness which was ravaging the Welsh borders, leaving Henry therefore as the legitimate successor to the throne.[1]

Immediately on the receipt of the tragic news, Catherine's parents—unwilling to abandon the diplomatic advantages offered by the marriage of their daughter to the English heir-apparent—started negotiations for the marriage of the young widow to her still younger brother-in-law. A marriage of this kind was of course forbidden both by earthly law and heavenly injunction; but fortunately a dispensation from the Pope was capable of overcoming both these obstacles. Henry's father too was not unwilling for the match: but a dispute arose over Catherine's dowry, part only of which had been paid. Ferdinand not only refused to pay the balance, but even demanded the return of the part already paid, while Henry VII on his side required the whole of the dowry as originally contemplated.

While the dispute was still in progress, Henry VII became a widower and thereupon proposed, as a fresh solution of the problem, that he himself should marry Catherine. Whether this proposal was an earnest one or not, it was certainly calculated to stir the Œdipus

---

[1] In later life Henry showed a very lively fear of the sweating sickness— a fear which has exposed him to a charge of cowardice at the hands of unfavourable historians. If, as seems to be the case, this fear was a somewhat isolated and unusual feature of his character, it would not seem unreasonable to suppose that its abnormal strength was due to the notion of a talion punishment—an idea often found in the unconscious levels of the mind : in other words, that Henry was afraid lest the same sickness which had unexpectedly swept away his rival (thus gratifying his desires of greatness) would in turn prove the means of his own undoing.

complex in young Henry's mind, by bringing him into a situation of such a kind that he could scarcely but regard himself as in some sense a sexual rival of his father, while at the same time it was likely to reinforce the transference of the mother-regarding feelings on to Catherine.

Whatever its ultimate psychological effects may have been, the proposal was undoubtedly successful as an immediate diplomatic measure. Ferdinand and Isabella moderated their terms with regard to the dowry: the marriage of brother and sister-in-law appeared eminently respectable as compared with the more shocking union of father and daughter-in-law, and the marriage treaty between young Henry and Catherine was definitely settled, it being arranged that the wedding should be celebrated as soon as Henry should have attained his fourteenth year.

But the death of Isabella shortly afterwards induced Henry VII to repent of this arrangement. There were various claimants for the crown of Castile and the whole political situation became for a time uncertain and obscure. The alliance with Ferdinand lost much of its attractiveness, a variety of fresh schemes for the marriage of young Henry were freely discussed and on the eve of his fifteenth birthday he solemnly repudiated the marriage contract which he had previously signed.

Three years later, however, in spite of various projects, no further betrothal had been made. Meanwhile Henry VII had reached the end of his career, and on his deathbed seems to have reverted to his original plan as regards the younger Henry's marriage. The dying king exhorted his son to complete the long-projected and much-delayed union with his sister-in-law, and gave at the same time sundry other pieces of advice, most of which Henry took well to heart. Indeed there can be but little doubt that a tendency to follow the expressed wishes of his dead father—a "postponed obedience" of the kind with which psycho-analysts are familiar—formed a by no means unimportant element in Henry's character during the earlier years of his reign. Among his other deathbed wishes Henry VII expressed the desire that his son should defend the Church, make war upon the Infidel, pay good heed to his faithful councillors, and (perhaps also) that he should put out of the way Edmund de la Pole, Earl of Suffolk, the nearest White Rose claimant to the throne. The troubled state of European politics prevented young Henry from making war on an extensive scale upon the Turk,[1] but the other behests he truly carried out. Henry, throughout his early years (and indeed in some sense throughout his life) was much concerned to preserve the true religion and the institution of the Church; both by his deeds and by his written words he fought against all doctrines and tendencies which he regarded as heretical. So great indeed was his ardour in this direction that he won from the spiritual head of Christendom the title of Defender of the Faith—a title borne by his successors to this day. With regard to councillors, his dependence on their approval and advice (and especially on that of Wolsey) in the first half of his reign is notorious; while de la Pole, imprisoned from the first, was executed four years afterwards.

If in these matters Henry obeyed the dying wishes

---

[1] It should be noted however :—(1) that his very first military undertaking was of this kind (the expedition of 1511 to co-operate with his *father-in-law* Ferdinand against the Moors) ; (2) that Henry declared that " he cherished like an heirloom the ardour against the Infidel which he inherited from his father," (A. F. Pollard, *Henry VIII*, p. 54).

of his father, he was no less willing to follow the latter's instructions as regards marriage, especially perhaps, in this case, because these instructions coincided with the tendencies emanating from his own unconscious Œdipus complex; enabling him in this way to combine a conscious obedience to the behests of filial piety with a realization of unconscious desires connected with hostility and jealousy towards his father and brother. The marriage was indeed hurried forward with almost indecent haste, being celebrated a little over a month after the elder Henry's death. A few days later the young couple were crowned King and Queen with much splendour and ceremony in Westminster Abbey.

Henry having now succeeded to the throne in his eighteenth year, a variety of circumstances combined to make his position in some ways an exceptional one in the whole history of English monarchy. He was the only surviving son of his father and it was generally recognized that in his person were bound up all hopes of freedom from internal discord. The Wars of the Roses were by now sufficiently distant to make the claims of other possible aspirants to the throne appear unsubstantial as compared with the firm *de facto* rights of the Tudor family, while at the same time the memory of those wars was still strong enough to make even a tyrannous exercise of royal power seem preferable to the alternative of civil war or anarchy. Added to these circumstances tending to make Henry's power as King more than usually absolute were other factors of a more personal nature. Henry possessed abilities and qualities unusual in degree and number and of such a kind as to make him as a prince intensely popular. All contemporary authorities agree in describing him as exceptionally handsome, tall, strong, skilful, and talented in arts and letters, with a very special degree of aptitude for all the manly sports and exercises of his age. Englishmen of the sixteenth century had in their way as much affection for a true "sportsman" as those of the nineteenth and twentieth centuries, and Henry's popularity with many of his subjects was, as one historian suggests,[1] probably not less than that which would at the present time fall to the lot of a young monarch who was a hero of the athletic world, "the finest oar, the best bat, the crack marksman of his day." Henry, moreover, was very fond of all kind of social festivity and merriment, delighting in sumptuous display and courtly ceremony—qualities which, though they eventually led to difficulties through the extravagance which they engendered, yet appeared at first a welcome contrast to the somewhat austere and parsimonious régime of his father.

This combination of happy circumstances may well have fostered in the young King an undue development of the positive self-regarding and self-seeking motives, the tendencies calculated to lead to such development being in his case greater even than are those to which most youthful rulers are exposed. Nevertheless, although fully conscious both of the prerogatives due to his circumstances and station and of his own personal abilities, he seldom (especially during the early part of his reign) became harsh, overbearing, tyrannous, or disrespectful of the advice or opinions of others. His self-reliance and self-will were happily tempered by a sound appreciation of the nature and extent of the forces—psychological and sociological—with which he had to deal, and by a certain piety and regard for

[1] Pollard, *op. cit.*, p. 41.

persons or bodies carrying the weight of constitutional or traditional authority.

Psycho-analysts will be inclined to regard this last characteristic as a displacement of tendencies and feelings originally directed to the person of his father. We have already seen some evidence of this in connection with the carrying out of his father's deathbed wishes. Henry's reliance on his councillors—Warham, Wolsey, Cromwell and others, his persistent desire to proceed in accordance with, rather than against, legal and constitutional authority, his anxiety to gain the approval of, and—later—to conciliate, the Pope, may all very probably be correctly regarded as further manifestations of this side of his character—a side which is of great importance for a true appreciation of his personality, and one which may easily be overlooked on a first casual view of his career.

These two sets of motives—the egoistic and the venerative we may perhaps, for the sake of brevity, be allowed to call them—through their conflicts, interactions and combinations probably played a very weighty rôle in determining Henry's conduct, and through this, of producing many of the outstanding features—political and domestic—of his reign. We shall have occasion to refer to them more than once in our examination of the subsequent events of his life.

To return now to the history of Henry's married life: the early years with Catherine seem to have been gay and happy. Only very gradually did Henry become dissatisfied and superstitious as regards the union with his sister-in-law. No doubt a variety of causes contributed to the eventual rupture, which did not begin till 1527—eighteen years after the celebration of the marriage. Catherine, in spite of some excellent qualities, was tactless, obstinate and narrow-minded, and had not that (real or apparent) pliability and subservience which Henry, in virtue of his egoistic tendencies, demanded in a consort. Worse than this, Catherine appears to have suffered from a father-fixation of some strength, as a result of which she was unable to transfer adequately her loyalty and affection from her parents and the land of her birth to her husband and the land of her adoption.[1] For many years she wrote to her father in the most pious and obedient terms, and regularly acted as his ambassador and the supporter of his interests—interests that often did not coincide with, and were sometimes in direct opposition to, those of her husband; while even in purely English affairs, she sometimes acted in a manner prejudicial to Henry's influence and desires.

The most important factor was, however, beyond doubt Catherine's inability to produce a male heir to the throne and the general unfruitfulness of the marriage, which from the point of view of issue was a long and almost unbroken series of disasters (due to miscarriages, premature and still births), the only surviving child being the Princess Mary, born in 1516. Henry's need of a legitimate son was a very real one. Without a recognized successor, the security of the throne and the kingdom was in danger, as there could be no doubt that in such a case there would arise at Henry's death many claimants for the supreme power. Henry, moreover, was peculiarly sensitive on this point. There can be little doubt that, like many others, he saw in

[1] It must be said however in Catherine's defence that the circumstances of Arthur's early death and of the none too flattering or considerate treatment that she received in England during the period of her young widowhood were certainly calculated to produce a regression of feeling in favour of her own family and home.

his heirs a continuation of his own life and power—
an immortalization of himself, without which his egoistic
impulses could find no complete satisfaction.

Furthermore, this failure in the fertility of his
marriage aroused superstitious fears connected with
Henry's Œdipus complex. The idea of sterility as a
punishment for incest is one that is deeply rooted in
the human mind,[1] and in the case of a union such as
that of Henry's and Catherine's, there was scriptural
authority for the infliction of a penalty of this description.[2] The scruples of conscience which were originally
urged as a reason for the delay in the marriage may
have been a mere diplomatic move on the part of Henry
VII, but in the case of the younger Henry, in view of
his genuine respect for religion and of the nature of
the unconscious feelings he entertained towards his
brother, they may well have had some real psychological foundation. Quieted for a time as the result of
his father's deathbed wishes and Henry's own inclinations, these scruples gradually rose again when the
course of events seemed to be bringing the divine
prophecy very near to fulfilment, and beyond all
reasonable doubt they constituted a genuine and all-
important factor in Henry's desire for a divorce from
Catherine. Brewer, as the result of a prolonged study
of contemporary documents, tells us that Henry's
doubts and fears upon this subject rose slowly in his
mind as the result of more or less unconscious processes.
"The exact date at which Henry began to entertain
these scruples and their precise shape at the first,

[1] See, for instance, Sir J. G. Frazer, *Totemism and Exogamy*, Vol. IV,
pp. 106 ff.

[2] " If a man shall take his brother's wife, it is an unclean thing. He
hath uncovered his brother's nakedness. They shall be childless." *Leviticus*
xx., 21.

can never be determined with accuracy; for the most sufficient of all reasons: they were not known to the king himself. They sprung up unconsciously from a combination of causes, and took definite form and colour in his breast by insensible degrees. They must have brooded in his mind some time before he would acknowledge them to himself, still less confess them to others."[1] Such gradual growth of feelings of this kind is totally opposed to the popular view that Henry's desire to divorce Catherine was merely an outcome of his sensual longing for Anne Boleyn, and indicates the operation of more deep-lying mental processes, such as those we have suggested, *i.e.* the arousal of fears resting on the repression of incestuous desires—desires in all probability originally connected with his parents (Œdipus complex), but, through the force of circumstances, transferred to his brother and sister-in-law.

This is not to say, of course, that Henry's attachment for Anne did not also play an important part in his desire to be rid of Catherine. Probably nothing else but a genuine passion for Anne would have kept him constant and inflexible during the long and difficult period of the divorce. Catherine was six years older than Henry, and the mental and physical strain attendant on her long and unsuccessful series of attempts at childbearing had no doubt considerably diminished her attractiveness. Before his infatuation with Anne Boleyn, Henry had enjoyed the favours of two mistresses:—Elizabeth Blount, by whom he had, so far as we know, his only illegitimate child—a boy— whom, with the failure of male heirs, he afterwards thought seriously of raising to the position of successor to the throne; and Mary Boleyn, sister of Anne Boleyn.

[1] *Reign of Henry VIII*, Vol. II, p. 162.

We know comparatively little of these affairs and the very existence of the second liaison has been sometimes doubted.[1]

By psycho-analysts, accustomed as they are to attach importance to apparently inessential details of this kind, it may not be considered unworthy of notice that the Christian names of the two ladies in question are the same as those held by important members of Henry's own family — his mother and younger sister respectively. The suspicion thus raised that the name may have been of some importance in determining Henry's choice in these two cases is strengthened by three further facts, which may be briefly mentioned here: (1) Henry's two daughters were also called by the same two names, viz. Mary and Elizabeth respectively; (2) his only other female favourite, whom we know by name, was Margaret Shelton, the Christian name being here identical with that of Henry's elder sister (wife of James IV of Scotland); (3) Mary Boleyn's mother was Lady *Elizabeth* Boleyn, and there existed a curious rumour that Henry had indulged in improper relations with the mother, as well as with the daughter.[2]

It is true that Henry is reported to have himself denied the truth of this; but even if (as is very possibly the case) the rumour itself is exaggerated, it may well have been founded on some genuine attraction which Henry may have felt for the Lady Elizabeth. If this is so, in the light of psycho-analytic knowledge, it would appear not overbold to suggest that the mother and daughter, Elizabeth and Mary Boleyn, were, to

---

[1] Though the proofs of its existence seem quite adequate. See Paul Friedmann, *Anne Boleyn*, Vol. II, Appendix B.

[2] Brewer, *Letters and Papers*, IV, CCCXXIX, footnote; also *Reign of Henry VIII*, Vol. II, p. 170; Friedmann, *op. cit.*, Vol. II, p. 326.

Henry's unconscious mind, substitutes for Elizabeth and Mary Tudor—his mother and his sister respectively. This would at once constitute additional evidence in favour of the existence in Henry of incest tendencies and family fixations and fit in with certain important features of Henry's relationship to Anne Boleyn, which are as follows:

One of the most inconsistent facts about the divorce of Catherine and subsequent marriage with Anne is that, although the incestuous relationship between Henry and Catherine was made the sole and all-important ground for claiming the divorce, the immediately succeeding second marriage involved the consummation of a relationship extremely similar to that which was supposed to invalidate the first. Catherine was Henry's sister in virtue of her previous marriage with his brother Arthur: Anne was his sister in virtue of his own (illicit) relationship to her sister Mary. He was therefore only giving up one sister in order to take another; and the very same (papal) powers that had to be invoked to grant the dissolution of the first marriage on the ground of incest had to be approached with a view to granting a dispensation because of the incestuous nature of the second union. Viewed in the light of sound diplomacy or of reasonable moral sense, the inconsistency involved in this procedure is absurdly evident. It cannot in fact be accounted for on either of these planes of thought. Such inconsistency, however, is quite a characteristic feature of conduct determined—partly or wholly—by unconscious complexes, and as such, probably, it has to be regarded and explained.

It is not necessary here to enter into the long and tedious history of the proceedings for divorce, which extended over a period of six years, from 1527 to 1533. These proceedings derive their great historical importance from the fact that they were the occasion of the breach with Rome (the breach that opened the way to the Reformation in England). Their importance for the development of Henry's mind and character is due to a similar reason. The main original difficulty in the granting of the divorce (apart from the very strong popular feeling in England in favour of Catherine) was due to the following facts:—first, it involved the annulling of the previous papal dispensation—a procedure which might seem liable to bring future papal dispensations (and indeed the papal power generally) into disrepute; secondly and chiefly, the Pope was at that time in the power of Charles V, who, both for political and family reasons—he was of course Catherine's nephew—was opposed to the divorce.

The Pope being thus, by the force of circumstances, brought into opposition with Henry's policy and unable to grant the divorce, as he had done recently in the case of other highly placed persons,[1] obstacles of one kind or another were continually placed in the way of Henry's desire. The consequent long delay in the realization of his wishes brought up in Henry's mind a conflict between the two aspects of his character to which we have previously referred—the egoistic and venerative aspects, with results of great importance, both for his future married life and his career in general. In virtue probably of the feelings of love and respect which he held towards his father, Henry was in his

---

[1] Notably in the case of Louis XII before he married Henry's sister Mary, in that of Brandon, Duke of Suffolk, previous to his marriage to the same sister after Louis's death and in that of Henry's other sister Margaret—cases which were certainly in Henry's mind as precedents.

early years most anxious to win and retain the approval of the Pope.[1] He had ever been willing to defend the Pope and the Church in word and deed, both against armed force and spiritual heresy, in fact "his championship of the Holy See had been the most unselfish part of Henry's policy;"[2] and there was no doubt that he was most anxious to obtain the quasi-paternal sanction of the divorce and re-marriage which a papal edict would afford.

But as time passed, and the inability to obtain the fulfilment of his desires with the Pope's consent and approval became more and more apparent, Henry's egoistic motives began to gain the mastery and to overwhelm the venerative tendencies, which had hitherto formed such an important element in his character. So far indeed did the former motives eventually prevail that Henry ultimately brought himself, not only to arrange for the divorce to be carried out at home without the Pope's authority, to defy at once the Pope, the Emperor and his own people and to brave the terrors of the papal excommunication, but even to set himself in the Pope's place by becoming the head of the Church in England and to assume a power, temporal and spiritual, which has never perhaps been equalled by any other British sovereign. This splendid triumph of self-assertion, in the face of severe obstacles [3] can only have been achieved

---

[1] The Pope of course, as his very title signifies, is one of the most regular and normal father substitutes.

[2] Pollard, *op. cit.*, p. 107.

[3] Cf. the words of Pollard, *op. cit.*, p. 306. " It was the King and the King alone, who kept England on the course which he had mapped out. Pope and Emperor were defied ; Europe was shocked ; Francis himself disapproved of the breach with the Church ; Ireland was in revolt ; Scotland, as ever, was hostile ; legislation had been thrust down the throats of a recalcitrant Church, and, we are asked to believe, of a no less unwilling House of Commons, while the people at large were seething with indignation at the insults heaped upon the injured Queen and her daughter."

by a very complete victory of the egoistic over the venerative tendencies. That such a victory took place is indicated by Henry's contempt of the power which he had formerly exalted, as when he said that "if the Pope issued ten thousand excommunications, he would not care a straw for them," that "he would show the Princes how small was really the power of the Pope" and "that when the Pope had done what he liked on his side, he (Henry) would do what he liked here." In such an attitude of defiance psycho-analysts will immediately recognize a displacement of the desire to overthrow the rule of the father and usurp his authority —a desire based on the primitive Œdipus complex.

From the time of his split with Rome, Henry's character underwent a marked transformation. He became vastly more despotic, determined to rule as well as to reign; more intolerant of any kind of limitation of his power, and dependent on his own decisions in all matters, great and small, instead of submitting to the advice of councillors, as he had hitherto so largely done.

The most significant and important step in this last direction was of course that which brought about the fall of Wolsey. It is fairly certain that, in the day of his power, Wolsey too was regarded by Henry with feelings originally connected with his father-venerative tendencies. These feelings may have flowed more freely and more consistently on to Wolsey's person because, as Friedmann well suggests,[1] Wolsey, as an ecclesiastic, was not brought into such direct competition with Henry's claims to manly qualities, as a layman would have been. The fields of war, sport and sex were, for instance, excluded, and the sphere

---

[1] *Op. cit.*, Vol. I, p. 34.

of politics, in which Wolsey so excelled, was one in which Henry only gradually began to take a lively interest. However, when this interest reached a certain degree of intensity, as it did under the stimulus of the proceedings for divorce, Henry became intolerant of Wolsey's guidance, with the inevitable result of Wolsey's fall.[1]

After Wolsey's fall none other attained his unique position; even Cromwell, in the height of his power, occupying a far inferior place. As regards religion too, Henry moved on a consistent road to power. In creating himself head of the Church, he not only took unto himself the paternal authority of the Pope, but became to some extent a sharer of the divine power of which the Pope had been the earthly representative. As Luther declared "Junker Henry meant to be God, and to do as pleased himself." [2]

This identification of himself with God—the God complex, as Ernest Jones has called it [3]—found further

---

[1] Though other important influences were also of course at work, notably :— (1) Wolsey's connection with the Church ; (2) the well-founded suspicion that Wolsey was not too favourably disposed to the projected marriage with Anne Boleyn, Wolsey thus becoming an obstacle to the consummation of Henry's sexual desires, and in this way bringing upon himself the hostile elements of Henry's Œdipus complex.

In his later dealings with Wolsey and with Warham, Archbishop of Canterbury, Henry would seem sometimes to have had in mind a comparison between his own relations to the Cardinal and the Archbishop and those of his predecessor, Henry II, to Thomas à Becket (*e.g.* Pollard, *op. cit.*, p. 271). It is noteworthy in this connection that, whereas during the early part of his career Henry was in the habit of showing his respect for the murdered archbishop by making a yearly offering at his shrine, in 1538 he added to his offences against the Church by despoiling the same shrine and burning the saintly bones, and is even said to have held a mock trial of the saint, who was condemned as a *traitor*.

[2] *Letters and Papers*, XVI, 106.

[3] "Der Gottmenschkomplex," *Zeitschrift für ärztliche Psychoanalyse*, 1913, I, p. 313. English translation : "The God Complex " in *Essays in Applied Psycho-Analysis*, p. 204.

R

expression in his breaking up of the monasteries, his prohibitions against the worship of saints and images, the consistent exclusion of clerics from the higher posts of state which they had hitherto occupied, and the endeavours to define the orthodox faith and produce — by force if necessary — a general uniformity of religious belief within his dominions: all measures tending to prevent the possibility of opposition or rivalry to his quasi-omnipotent power in the religious sphere.

Throughout all this magnificent triumph of the egoistic tendencies, Henry steered his course with a level head. His success in the face of circumstances which would have been the undoing of most other monarchs was due partly to the unique conditions of his time, which, as we have seen, made possible and even agreeable a degree of despotism which at other periods would have been resented; partly, to the exceeding strength of will and self-reliance that Henry developed after the overthrow of the father-regarding venerative attitude in the course of his struggle with the Pope; partly, too, to his firm grasp of reality in the field of politics. Few men have been able to reconcile, as he did, an intense egotism and an enormous lust for power with an undistorted vision of forces and events; and in the unique degree to which he achieved this combination is probably to be sought the ultimate secret of his political success.

The divorce of Catherine, which had provided the occasion for this gradual but momentous change in Henry's character, was after many delays and vicissitudes, eventually hurried forward to a rapid conclusion by the fact of Anne having become pregnant and the consequent necessity of legalizing her relationship to Henry, if her child (supposing it should be a son) was to become the recognized heir to the throne. In spite of Henry's long infatuation for Anne, he had not succeeded in making her his mistress till towards the end of 1532. Warned perhaps by the somewhat fickle nature of Henry's affection for his previous mistresses, Anne determined to avoid the consummation of her intimacy with the King, and kept her resolution until the success of the divorce seemed certain.

Subsequent events amply demonstrated the wisdom of this delay on her part. She was married to Henry in January, 1533, and in the following May Henry was already beginning to grow tired of her. Though steadfast in his affections for years in the face of difficulties, as soon as all obstacles were removed and he had full and unquestioned possession of her whom he had so long desired, Henry's love began to cool and he became conscious of defects in Anne of which he had previously been unobservant. Here we see clearly for the first time the manifestation of what seems to have been a very important trait of Henry's sexual life, viz. that there was usually some impediment in the way of the free expression of his love towards the women of his choice. In Anne's case the impediment lay doubtless to some extent in her refusal to give herself up fully to her royal lover until she became certain that she would be his consort rather than his mistress. But there were deeper underlying factors connected with the very circumstance of the love having been previously illicit—a circumstance which gave it an attraction that a legalized union failed to possess.

In an illuminating paper on the varieties of the love life [1] Freud has shown that the need for an obstacle to

---

[1] Beiträge zur Psychologie des Liebeslebens, *Jahrbuch für psychoanalytische und psychopathologische Forschungen*, 1910, II, p. 389.

be present as a condition for the arousal of love can be traced back to the operation of the Œdipus complex. In the earliest love of a boy for his mother such an obstacle is constituted by the incestuous nature of the relationship. Furthermore, the mother, as the object of the boy's love, is already bound by ties of law and affection to a third person, the father. In a number of cases where the psycho-sexual development has not been carried far enough to ensure adequate freedom from the infantile fixation on the parents, the continued existence of the Œdipus complex manifests itself in the choice of a love-object, between whom and the lover there is an impediment of the kind that existed in the original incestuous love; *i.e.* either the love itself is unlawful or the loved object is already bound elsewhere, or else (as often happens) both conditions are present. Now there can be little doubt that Henry was a person whose Œdipus complex found expression in such a way. On this hypothesis it becomes possible to explain two very constant features of his love life: his fickleness (which made him unable to love a woman, once his possession of her was assured) and the desire for some obstacle between him and the object of his choice. We shall come across sufficient examples of these, as we study the further course of his chequered conjugal career.

The facts connected with the fall of Anne Boleyn show more clearly than any other event, not only the existence of a desire for an impediment of this kind, but the foundation of this desire in an incestuous fixation. At the same time they give the key to a true understanding of the central conflict involved in Henry's sexual life—that " common cause " of Henry's matrimonial difficulties, which, as Froude says, " ought to be discoverable." Henry, as we saw, soon tired of Anne after his marriage with her. The fact that her child, born in 1533, was a daughter (the future Queen Elizabeth), instead of the long-desired male heir, only served still further to alienate Henry's affections. During the three years of his married life with Anne, Henry consoled himself, first with some lady whose name does not seem to have come down to us, then with Margaret Shelton, and finally with Jane Seymour, his future wife, who appears to have aroused his genuine love. The thought of putting Anne aside seems to have been present for some considerable period before it was put into execution, matters being delayed for a time by the fact that a repudiation of Anne might have necessitated a return to Catherine.

Catherine's death in January 1536 (hurried on, as some think, by means of poison) removed this difficulty, and Anne's miscarriage (probably her second) in the same month served to revive the scruples with regard to incest that Henry had already experienced in relation to his first marriage. These scruples, which on their first arousal had grown slowly and by insensible degrees, now quickly regained their mastery over Henry's mind. The union with his second sister-representative (Anne) was now as repellent to him, on account of its incestuous flavour, as had been that with his first sister-representative (Catherine). Anne was accused of having been unfaithful to her husband, quite a number of persons being charged as her accomplices, and of having been repeatedly guilty of incest with her brother, Lord Rochford. She was further accused of having conspired with her lovers to bring about the death of the King and of having, through her treasonable behaviour, so injured his health as to put his life in danger. All the more important male prisoners concerned in these charges were found guilty of high treason and were put to death, Anne herself following them to the scaffold a few days later.

At the same time her marriage with Henry was declared invalid, probably on one or more of the following grounds:[1]—(1) the existence of an alleged precontract with the Earl of Northumberland; (2) the affinity between Anne and Henry arising from the latter's relations with Mary Boleyn. The very day after Anne's death, Henry was married to Jane Seymour.

Historians are pretty generally agreed that (although Anne was far from being incapable of loose living or even of more serious offences) there was as a matter of fact little or no truth in any of the long series of grave charges brought against her. In particular there seems to be no satisfactory evidence at all in favour of the charges of incest and of treason. We are therefore free to regard these accusations as for the most part reflections of Henry's own mental state, for although Cromwell and others were responsible for the details of the matter, "Henry was regularly informed of every step taken against Anne and her associates and interfered a good deal with the proceedings," and "his wishes probably influenced the form in which the indictments were drawn up."[2]   His interest in the proceedings and their psychological significance for him is further shown by the fact that he composed a tragedy on the subject, which he showed to the Bishop of Carlisle at a gay supper very shortly after Anne's execution.[3]

In accusing Anne of incest with her brother, Henry

[1] See Pollard, *op. cit.*, p. 344.   [2] Friedmann, *op. cit.*, Vol. II, p. 268.
[3] Friedmann, *op. cit.*, Vol. II, p. 267.

produced with reference to his brother-in-law a repetition of the situation which had formerly existed as between himself and his own brother in the case of Catherine. In both cases he was (in reality or in imagination) brought into competition with his brother over the person of his sister. The circumstances under which he had first been brought into rivalry with his brother Arthur (calculated, as these were, to arouse in a slightly altered form the original Œdipus complex)[1] had, it would appear, made so firm an impression on his psycho-sexual tendencies and dispositions, that he continued to desire a repetition of the situation under which his sexual impulses had first been aroused.

But the feelings called forth by his relations to Arthur and Catherine were ambivalent in character, as is almost invariably the case with those connected with the Œdipus complex and its displacements. On the one hand there was the desire to kill his brother (father-substitute) and marry his sister (mother-substitute), while at the same time there was also present a horror of these things. In the long period of Catherine's divorce, it was of course the horror that was uppermost in Henry's conscious mind; but simultaneously the attractiveness of incest manifested itself in the choice of a fresh sister-substitute in the person of Anne—giving rise to that strange contradiction in Henry's behaviour of which we have already spoken. After a time (shortened, it would appear, by Anne's miscarriages, which aroused Henry's previous superstitions) the negative attitude

[1] It must not be forgotten that the facts of his parents being within the forbidden degrees of affinity and of their requiring a papal dispensation, just as he himself did later on, were doubtless known to Henry and thus probably constituted a strong associative link between his parents' marriage and his own union with Catherine ; another link being formed probably by his father's proposal to marry Catherine after Arthur's death.

to incest was transferred in turn to his relations with Anne. In the hatred of Anne which was thus occasioned Henry *projected* on to her his own incestuous desires; *i.e.* he accused her of incestuous relations with her brother, whereas the real fact was that Henry himself desired incestuous relations with his sister. In this way Henry was able to enjoy by proxy the fulfilment of his own repressed desires, while at the same time giving expression to his horror and disgust at the relationship concerned.

By the same means too he was able to provide an outlet for the jealousy, fear and hatred he felt towards his brother. Just as Henry himself had, through the accident of Arthur's death, inherited the throne in place of his brother, so now he seems to have feared that his own place in turn would be usurped by a brother. Hence the charge of treason, for which there appears to be even less evidence than for the supposed sexual offences, and which therefore, to the psychoanalyst, reveals clearly enough the circumstance that, although Henry was not in fact guilty of Arthur's death, he nevertheless felt guilty on the subject, since the death constituted a realization of his own repressed desires.[1]

By a process familiar to the student of unconscious mental life, the brother rôle seems to have been filled in Henry's phantasy by more than one person at this time. The sexual aspects of the part were of course taken principally (but not entirely) by Anne's brother, Rochford; but the accusations of treason were directed more especially against one, Henry Noreys, who was

---

[1] Here again the brother enmity was probably only a displacement of the earlier father enmity, for, as we have seen above, Henry had in some respects, special grounds for imagining himself in his father's place.

supposed to have arranged to marry Anne after Henry's death. Noreys appears to have been the only one of the accused whom Henry honoured with a personal interview on the subject of his misdemeanours and whom he privately urged to confession.[1] Now it is suggestive that shortly before this incident Noreys has acquired a quasi-personal relationship to Henry by becoming betrothed to Margaret Shelton, who had quite recently been Henry's favourite and probably his mistress. In view of the fact that much emphasis was laid on Anne's becoming a sister of Henry's in virtue of his relations to Mary Boleyn, it would seem not unlikely that, by a similar process of thought, Noreys might be regarded as Henry's brother in virtue of his betrothal to Margaret. If any such process did take place in Henry's mind, the reason for the special charges against Noreys and the special attention paid to him by Henry is to a great extent explained.[2]

In order to prevent the recurrence of such schemes as had been attributed to Anne and Noreys, Henry had resort to legislation. By a clause in the Act of Succession (an act passed primarily to declare Anne's daughter Elizabeth a bastard and to settle the crown on Henry's prospective issue by Jane) it was made high treason for anyone to marry a King's daughter, sister or aunt without royal permission—a measure by which Henry would appear to have tried to do away once and for all with the fear of sexual rivals in his own family.

We have seen how, during the divorce of Catherine, while the negative (horror) aspect of the incest complex

---

[1] Friedmann, op. cit., Vol. II, p. 251.

[2] It is just possible too that, as perhaps in other cases, the name *Henry* may have been of some importance, referring of course to the Œdipus complex in its original (parent-regarding) form.

was in the ascendant towards Catherine herself, the positive (love) aspect was at the same time active in respect of Anne, so that, while Henry was getting rid of an incestuous relation with one sister, he was actually engaged in starting a fresh relation of the same kind with another sister. A very similar state of affairs seems to have arisen just before the fall of Anne. Undeterred by the result of his two preceding incestuous adventures, Henry was again contemplating marriage with a woman who was within the forbidden degrees of blood relationship. Jane Seymour "was descended on her mother's side from Edward III, and Cranmer had to dispense with a canonical bar to the marriage arising from her consanguinity to the King in the third and fourth degrees."[1] Although the actual relationship between Henry and Jane was thus relatively remote, it is probable that Henry's fancy saw in Jane a relative of a nearer kind; for, shortly before their marriage, he was in the habit of meeting her in the rooms of her *brother*, Sir Edward Seymour, whom he thus made as it were, a participant in the affair[2]— in this way endeavouring once more to re-establish the original brother-sister triangle.[3]

The circumstances connected with the fall of Anne Boleyn thus afford very clear evidence of two leading tendencies in Henry's psycho-sexual life — both of them conditioned by the facts of Henry's early love experiences, and through them by the still earlier Œdipus complex. These tendencies are:—(1) the desire for (and hatred of) a sexual rival; (2) the attrac-

---

[1] Pollard, *op. cit.*, p. 346.

[2] And who, it appears, had moved into these rooms (to which Henry had access by a secret passage) expressly for this purpose, the rooms having been previously occupied by Cromwell.

[3] Friedmann, *op. cit.*, Vol. II, p. 222.

tion towards (and at the same time the horror of) an incestuous relationship.

The same period gives us the first unmistakable indications of a third tendency (one intimately connected with the other two) which was henceforward to be of great importance, viz. Henry's insistence on chastity in his consort. We have already seen that his passion for Anne Boleyn seemed to be maintained in its original strength over a considerable number of years, to some extent at least because she refused to allow Henry the intimate privileges of her person. The same means were employed with equal effect by her successor Jane Seymour in the early days of her intimacy with Henry. So great was her assumption of virtue that she even refused presents from the King, because of their possible implication—a course which called forth much approval and admiration from Henry himself. While she thus made great show of chastity to Henry, there is reason to believe that she was not always as careful of her honour as she professed to be. Indeed some of Henry's contemporaries seem to have taken the view that Henry was more or less wilfully shutting his eyes to certain (probably well-known) facts in Jane's past history, facts of which he might afterwards become well aware, should it suit his purpose. Thus Chapuys, the ambassador of Charles V and a friend of Jane's, says in a letter written in May 1536: "She (Jane) is a little over twenty-five. You may imagine whether, being an Englishwoman, and having been so long at court, she would not hold it a sin to be still a maid. At which the King will perhaps be rather pleased . . . for he may marry her on condition that she is a virgin, and when he wants a divorce he will find plenty of witnesses to the contrary."[1]

[1] Quoted in Friedmann, *op. cit.*, Vol. II, p. 200.

In the light both of psychological knowledge and of later events (particularly those connected with Catherine Howard), it is probable that the inconsistency here involved was not altogether wilful or deliberate. It is more likely that we have to do with the manifestations of a conflict in Henry's mind—a conflict similar to those connected with the desire for a sexual rival and for an incestuous relationship, and leading, as in their case, to an inconsistent, fluctuating and ambivalent attitude. In fact there would appear to have existed two opposing motives; in virtue of the first Henry desired the most scrupulous chastity on the part of his wives, while at the same time, in virtue of the second, he secretly (and probably unconsciously) delighted in a partner who had already enjoyed sexual experience with other men, or who was actually unfaithful after marriage.

The explanation of this attitude is to be found, as before, in the facts connected with the Œdipus complex.[1] To the young boy the idea of sexual relations between the parents is apt to be a very disagreeable one. Jealousy of the father, the necessity of dissociating the parents from sexual thoughts (in order to surmount the stage of incestuous fixation), and a number of other potent factors, into which it is unnecessary to enter here, frequently give rise to the phantasy that no sexual relations exist or have existed between the parents— a phantasy that finds its supreme expression in the notion of the Virgin Mother and the Virgin Birth, which plays such a prominent part in religion, myth and legend. Now since, in later life, the wife is often unconsciously identified with the mother, it is not surprising that the ideas concerning chastity, originally

[1] Cp. Freud, *op. cit.*

aroused in connection with the latter, should be displaced on to the former: hence, in large measure the attraction which virginity exercises over many men.

On the other hand, the boy may soon discover or suspect the occurrence of sexual relations between his parents; and the having of such relations (in the past or in the present) may come to be regarded as an essential characteristic of the mother; and therefore any substitute for her in later life may be expected to exhibit the same characteristic, so that, in so far as the wife represents a mother surrogate, only women who have already enjoyed sexual experience are eligible for the position: hence, to some extent the fascination of widows.[1]

Now it would seem probable that in Henry's unconscious mind both these (mutually incompatible) notions of the mother had found a place, and that in the conflict between them we have the key to the inconsistency of his conduct in this respect.[2]

Having now arrived at a definite conception of the nature of the chief unconscious mental factors which

[1] By a further peculiar mental process, the mother will not infrequently come to be regarded as a prostitute, or at least as one who is very free with her favours. (Cp. Freud, *op. cit.*) Such an extension of the phantasy may very well have taken place in Henry's case, and would help to account for the *numerous* accusations of infidelity in the case of Anne Boleyn (only one of the accused men subsequently pleaded guilty and even the fact of his guilt has been doubted) and for the overlooking for so long a time of the rather openly promiscuous life led by Catherine Howard both before and after marriage.

[2] To the existence of these notions in Henry's mind was probably due much of the importance that was attached (during the divorce proceedings against Catherine of Aragon) to the question as to whether Catherine's marriage with Arthur had or had not been consummated. Catherine herself stated at a comparatively late stage of the proceedings that there had been no consummation, and in so doing she may have hoped to touch Henry at a point on which she knew him to be sensitive.

were operative in Henry's married life, we may content ourselves with a rapid examination of their influence on the remaining part of his career. His union with Jane Seymour was not destined to be of long duration. Jane died in October 1537, one year and four months after her marriage, and a few days after she had given birth to a son (afterwards Edward VI). Henry seems to have had throughout some genuine attachment to her, and she and Catherine Parr share the honour of being the only two of Henry's six wives who completed their conjugal career without a rupture. Possibly the brevity of this career in Jane's case may have prevented the occurrence of an alienation of Henry's affections such as Chapuys had anticipated (in the letter quoted above). Furthermore, the fact that she had presented him with the long-wished-for male heir probably added considerably to the warmth of Henry's feelings towards her. At any rate Henry seems to have cherished her memory for some considerable time, and at his own death, ten years after Jane's, accorded her the signal honour of being laid to rest in her tomb at Windsor.

During the period between Jane's death and Henry's eventual marriage with Anne of Cleves, his fourth wife, in 1539, various projects of marriage were discussed, none of which were destined to come to fruition, but in which the workings of Henry's unconscious tendencies can still to some extent be traced. The most important of these projects was connected with *Mary*, Duchess of Longueville, better known as Mary of Guise. Mary was *already affianced to Henry's nephew*, James V of Scotland (the desire for a rival and the tendency to incest—cp. too the name in this connection—both therefore being manifested in this case); but Henry insisted that the importance of his own

proposal ought to outweigh that of the previous arrangement. Francis I refused, however, to offend his ally
James by acceding to Henry's demand, and proposed
as a substitute Mary of Bourbon, daughter of the Duke
of Vendôme. Henry, however, rejected her forthwith,
on hearing that her hand had already been refused by
James (absence of attraction where there is no rivalry);
the two younger sisters of Mary of Guise were then
suggested, together with a number of other ladies at
the French court; and Henry, growing impatient and
irritated, demanded that a selection of the handsomest
available beauties should be sent to Calais for his
personal inspection and eventual choice. Francis,
however, rebelled against this scheme for "trotting out
the young ladies like hackneys," and the whole idea of
a French marriage was thereupon abandoned.

Meanwhile negotiations of a similar kind had been
started in the Netherlands. The lady here selected was
Christina, daughter of the deposed King of Denmark.
Christina had been married at a very early age to the
Duke of Milan and after a brief married life was now
a widow of sixteen—circumstances that recall vividly
those of Catherine of Aragon after Arthur's death.
For political reasons, however, the match was not
concluded and Henry was still without a wife.

Francis I and Charles V were at this time united in
friendship, and their alliance made Henry look for
support elsewhere, as a means of counterbalancing
their power. The Protestant princes of Germany
suggested themselves for this purpose. Religious
difficulties for some time barred the way, but in the
person of the Duke of Cleves Henry encountered one
whose policy was a compromise between Protestantism
and Romanism rather similar to that which he himself

adopted.[1] A match between Henry and Anne, the daughter of the Duke, was arranged, largely through Cromwell's influence, though an obstacle was present in the fact that Anne had been already promised to the son of the Duke of Lorraine. Though this fact may, here as elsewhere, have been an attraction to Henry, he seems on the whole to have behaved with remarkable passivity as regards the marriage. But a short time before he had said with reference to his contemplated French marriage, "I trust to no one but myself. The thing touches me too near. I wish to see them and know them some time before deciding." Now, however, he agreed to accept Anne on no better assurances than Cromwell's praises of her beauty and Holbein's none too flattering portrait. Perhaps he was willing to put an end at any cost to the worries of wife-hunting; perhaps too he was genuinely alarmed at the threatening political situation, for the Pope, the Emperor, and the Kings of France and Scotland were all arrayed against him and an invasion of England seemed not unlikely. Whatever the reason, he was very pliable in Cromwell's hands and even after he had seen and disapproved of Anne (whose appearance was homely, whose accomplishments were small when judged by the standard of the English and French courts, and who could speak no language but her own), he nevertheless consented to proceed with the marriage, distasteful as it was to him.

It was destined, however, to be the shortest of all his matrimonial ventures. In a few months the political situation had changed. Henry no longer needed the Protestant alliance, and lost no time in freeing himself from the *mariage de convenance* which had been entered

---

[1] Cp. Pollard, *op. cit.*, p. 383.

into with that end in view. In the summer of 1540 Cromwell, who had engineered the match and the alliance, was arrested and beheaded; while at the same time Henry's marriage with Anne was declared null and void, Henry pleading that he had not been a free agent in the matter, that Anne had never been released from her contract with the son of the Duke of Lorraine, that he (Henry) had only gone through the ceremony on the assumption that a release would be forthcoming and that consequently, actuated by a conscientious scruple, he had refrained from consummating the marriage.

Superficial as these reasons may well seem (for there is no doubt that Henry really wished to dissolve the match because Anne was unattractive to him—of which fact indeed he made no secret—and because the alliance for which the marriage stood was no longer necessary), it will be observed that they nevertheless bear unmistakable traces of Henry's unconscious tendencies, showing that these tendencies were active in this case also.[1]

Anne of Cleves being thus put out of the way, Henry immediately entered into a fifth marriage, with a lady to whose charms he had already fallen a victim—Catherine Howard, a niece of the Duke of Norfolk. For about a year and a half Henry lived with his new bride more happily perhaps than with any other of his consorts. He congratulated himself that "after sundry troubles of mind which had happened to him by marriage" he had at last found a blissful solution of

---

[1] Henry had previously complained to Cromwell that he suspected Anne (groundlessly, so far as we know) of being " no true maid "—thus showing the operation of the chastity complex as well as that connected with the presence of a rival.

S

his matrimonial difficulties; and in his chapel he returned solemn thanks to Heaven for the felicity which his conjugal state afforded him, directing his confessor, the Bishop of Lincoln, to compose a special form of prayer for that purpose.

This spell of happiness, however, was built on a delusion, Catherine Howard had lived anything but a chaste life before her marriage, though the king seems to have closed his eyes to the fact, as he had probably done before on a similar occasion. Even after her marriage, Catherine continued to receive her former lovers, particularly one Culpepper, to whom she had been previously affianced. Reports of the Queen's misconduct reached the ears of Cranmer, who with much trepidation brought the facts to Henry's knowledge. The latter at first refused to believe the charges, but, on the evidence becoming too strong to be resisted, was overwhelmed with surprise, grief, shame and anger, wept bitterly in public and generally manifested such emotion that "it was thought he had gone mad." He at first contemplated granting Catherine a pardon, but, on further proofs of quite recent misdemeanours coming to light, she was executed, together with her lovers and all those who had been her accomplices in one way or another.

We have here another very clear example of the working of Henry's unconscious complexes. Bearing in mind the great importance which he was wont to attach to virginity and chastity, together with the marked dissoluteness of Catherine's life and the comparatively little care she took to conceal it, it would seem that Henry was guilty of an almost pathological blindness in remaining ignorant of the true circumstances for so long. That there was indeed some definite repression at work is indicated too by his inability or unwillingness to believe the facts when they were first brought to his notice, and by his very great emotion on finally realizing the truth.

The mental forces here at work are, of course, those with which we are already familiar. On the one hand, Henry, as we have seen, desired a woman who had other lovers besides himself, while on the other hand he ardently desired her exclusive possession and her chastity. The conflict between these incompatible longings produced a temporary dissociation. For a time Henry was able to enjoy Catherine as if her dissoluteness and her infidelity did not exist—his enjoyment being indeed probably heightened by the very fact of her loose living, though the knowledge of her conduct in this respect was excluded from his conscious mind. When this knowledge did at length enter consciousness, he was overcome by his feelings, in much the same way as the bringing to light of unconscious factors in the course of psycho-analysis will often give rise to an emotional crisis.[1]

As he had done after the fall of Anne Boleyn, so now also, Henry resorted to legislative measures to prevent a recurrence of the disaster that had befallen him. On the previous occasion it had been made high treason to marry any woman nearly related to the King

---

[1] The emotion itself was probably complex both in nature and origin. From the accounts we have of his conduct, we may surmise that there were present, among other constituents : (1) grief, at the breakdown of his delusion —his happy life with Catherine being brought to a sudden and disastrous end ; (2) shame, both because he dimly realized that in the past his enjoyment had been largely due to gratification of forbidden desires (connected with the Œdipus complex) and because he had been made to look foolish before others ; (3) anger, directed both against Catherine and her accomplices for having deceived him and against himself for having allowed himself to be deceived.

S *

without the King's consent. The present enactments were primarily directed against female, rather than against male, offenders (following perhaps a development of Henry's mind, in virtue of which the chastity *motif* had been for some time increasing in importance), and it was declared treason for any woman to marry the King, if her previous life had not been strictly virtuous.

The new measure seems to have aroused considerable interest and amusement both in court and country, for the long series of Henry's matrimonial misadventures had now assumed to his contemporaries much the same laughable and yet tragic aspect which they still possess for us. In view of the strictness of the qualifications now required for the post of Queen, Chapuys suggested that "few, if any, ladies now at court will henceforth aspire to such an honour;"[1] while Henry's subjects, with a true appreciation both of his psychological needs and of the course of action to which these needs would impel him, jokingly remarked that only a widow would be able to meet the king's demands, as no reputed maid would ever be persuaded to incur the penalty of the statute.[2]

So indeed it actually turned out. In the early summer of 1543 Henry married Catherine Parr, his sixth and last wife. Although only thirty-one years of age, Catherine was then in her second widowhood—her second husband, Lord Latimer, having died at the end of 1542. In thus espousing one the fact of whose widowhood was especially striking, Henry was adopting the best compromise between his own conflicting tendencies and emotions. Catherine was chaste (her

---

[1] *Letters and Papers*, XVII, 124.

[2] And certainly, as we are now in a position to see, no sagacious woman would have done so; for however pure her past life might in reality have been, Henry would probably sooner or later have been impelled by his unconscious complexes to rake up some accusation of unchastity against her.

moral character was beyond reproach) and yet she had undoubtedly enjoyed previous sexual experience—a circumstance which, as we have seen, was necessary for the gratification of Henry's unconscious desires. At the same time another circumstance connected with Catherine Parr enabled Henry to satisfy to a large extent his other complexes. After the death of her second husband, Catherine's hand was sought by Sir Thomas Seymour *Henry's brother-in-law* (younger brother of Jane Seymour) to whom she appears to have been sincerely attached (and whom she eventually married after Henry's death—thus being, as Pollard says, "almost as much married as Henry himself"). Henry, however, overruled the engagement—in much the same way as he had attempted to do in the case of Mary of Guise—and compelled Catherine to abandon her lover in favour of himself.

The circumstances of Henry's last marriage thus strongly recall those connected with his first. The name of his bride was the same in both cases,[1] and in both cases he took the place which would otherwise have been filled by a brother. We thus see how the unconscious jealousy of Arthur (a jealousy which was itself probably only a displacement of that originally directed against his father) operated to the end of Henry's matrimonial career and acted as the determining factor in the choice of a wife more than forty years after Arthur's death. At the same time Catherine Howard's betrothal to Seymour in one sense constituted her a sister to Henry, so that the desire for an incestuous union was also satisfied.

A marriage entered into, as this one was, as the result

[1] The name may of course very well have been significant in the case of Catherine Howard also.

of a satisfactory compromise between the opposing forces of Henry's mind (all Henry's primitive unconscious desires rooted in the Œdipus complex finding gratification, but none of them too blatantly) gave promise of greater permanency and stability than did his previous ventures in matrimony: nor was this promise belied by the course of subsequent events. On one occasion, it is true, Catherine was in danger through having come into conflict with Henry's egoistic tendencies (which had become less and less restrained as he grew older), but her tact enabled her to surmount all difficulties arising from this source, and the marriage seems to have remained a happy one until Henry's death three and a half years later, in January 1547.

We have now traced the operation of certain unconscious motives throughout the whole of Henry's sexual life. For the sake of clearness we have distinguished three principal such motives: (1) a desire for opposition and the presence of a sexual rival, (2) a desire for incest, (3) a desire for chastity in his sexual partner. All these motives are closely interconnected, and they are all dependent on, and derived from, the primitive Œdipus complex; each motive, moreover, is present both in a positive and in a negative form. That which Henry was impelled to do by the operation of his unconscious desires he was equally impelled to oppose by the operation of (an often equally unconscious) resistance to these desires. Regarded as the outcome of the interaction of these various conflicting forces, the abnormal features of Henry's married life can, it would appear, very largely be explained.

The importance of studies such as that upon which we have been here engaged, apart from such value as they may have for the elucidation of historical problems, lies in the confirmation which they afford of results obtained by the process of psycho-analysis carried on with living individuals. These results are often so opposed to what we are accustomed to regard both as common sense and common decency, that their accept-ance is a matter of very considerable difficulty in the case of all persons who have not extensively employed the psycho-analytic method. Even to psycho-analysts themselves additional evidence for the validity of their conclusions from a fresh field of inquiry must always be most welcome. As such a source of additional evidence, the data of history would seem in some respects to be peculiarly acceptable. Although these data must always be inferior in scope and detail to evidence obtained from living persons, they present the following two great advantages: first, that the full data are open to investigation and verification by others, whereas in most psycho-analytic investigations the complete material on which conclusions are based are available only to the analyst himself; and secondly, that in the case of persons long since dead there can be no question of the influence either of direct sugges-tion or of the more subtle effects of psycho-analytic training and tradition. The actions and sayings of historical personages can have no possible reference to Freud's theories, whereas the patient in the physician's consulting-room is, it may be said, necessarily to some extent affected by the atmosphere of belief in psycho-analytic doctrine in which he finds himself.

Thus it would appear that the application of psycho-analytic findings to historical material[1] should furnish

---

[1] As of course to all records of human life and labour which have come about independently of the work of psycho-analysts themselves ; such as myths, legends, customs, literary and artistic productions, etc.

in general a most necessary and desirable test of the validity of the psycho-analytic method itself. If the psychic mechanisms revealed by the process of psycho-analysis upon the living subject are to be regarded as fundamental features of the human mind, and not as mere artifacts or pathological conditions occurring only in neurotic persons, they should be discoverable as factors operating in the lives of men and women of the past, wherever the available data bearing on these lives are adequate in quantity and quality. A certain number of studies directed to this end have already been made, and, by their demonstration of the fact that the behaviour of individuals long since dead can be satisfactorily accounted for on psycho-analytic theories (and perhaps in no other way), have afforded very valuable corroboration of the utility and validity of the psycho-analytic method. In the present paper we have endeavoured, it is hoped not altogether fruitlessly, to bring to light some further evidence pointing to the same conclusion.

INDEX